MENIERE MAN
AND THE GENIUS

THE MENIERE ANSWER BOOK

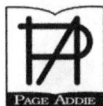

PAGE ADDIE PRESS
UNITED KINGDOM

Copyright

Contents

Learn from yesterday, live for today, hope for tomorrow. The important thing is not to stop questioning.

- Albert Einstein

INTRODUCTION

If you have opened this book right now on Meniere's, it is for one of three reasons. You have been diagnosed with Meniere's disease and want answers, or you know someone that is suffering and want to help. Or, like Albert Einstein, you know the importance of asking questions. This book is dedicated to answering questions about Meniere's disease.

When you are diagnosed with Meniere's disease, you have a lot of questions. And if you are lucky enough, you might come across a few people who have the same questions and luckier still, you'll receive exactly the answers you are looking for. Little did I know, that I'd be the one answering questions and sharing my feelings from a survivor's perspective.

You see, at the time I was diagnosed with Meniere's, I wasn't given any hope of making a recovery. Instead, I was handed a very simple A4 leaflet. All the specialist told me was to walk away from stress, and avoid salt. I knew no one who had suffered with Meniere's, let alone someone to talk to who had come out the other side as a Meniere's survivor.

Given no hope or information, Meniere's made me look inside myself, and in the process, I made discoveries about Meniere's and about myself. Over the years of doing talks and private mentoring, I realized most sufferers have the same worries and questions as I had. No matter how much they knew, they had similar questions. The main question everyone asks is how did Meniere Man get better? The answer to that important question is always the same. My recovery began with a decision. That decision was simply to get better. All my actions from that point on were about working towards recovery. I knew the direction I was going. I worked through Meniere's disease, figured out about triggers, diet, exercise, stress, medication, meditation, and shunned options for surgical intervention. Then, contrary to my prognosis, I made a complete recovery. Working through the condition gave me the right experience to share what I believe helped my recovery.

I wrote self-help books on Meniere's disease to help others who were interested in adopting a positive attitude to make Meniere's less of a hindrance, improve one's lifestyle, and go on to ultimately have a normal life, free of Meniere's. Dealing with Meniere's does require patience, a strong will and hard work to succeed, and overcome. It isn't easy, but there's a way to re-frame everything. Think of this book as a tool to help you understand and explore Meniere's. It may also stimulate other questions you may wish to discuss with your doctor, and specialist. Meniere's disease is manifold and so no one person can have all of the answers.

Answers to questions are an essential step to wellness. questions, like 'Can I die from Meniere's?'

The answer is categorically NO!

Raising questions is an important part of coming to terms with a medical condition. As in the book of life, the answers are not at the back end.

ON THE QUESTION OF MENIERE'S DISEASE

Q: What kind of Meniere's disease did you have?

A: After undergoing a series of tests to rule out any other physical cause, I was diagnosed with classic (typical) Meniere's disease.

Q: What symptoms did you have for classic Meniere's?

A: I had four specific symptoms: Episodic fluctuating rotational vertigo (spinning). Episodic and fluctuating tinnitus (a sound heard when there is no sound). Episodic and fluctuating aural fullness (a sensation of pressure in the ear). Episodic and fluctuating hearing loss.

Q: How do you pronounce Meniere's?

A: \men-'yerz-

Q: Is Meniere's disease hereditary?

A: While Meniere's disease is not genetic or hereditary, the incidence is slightly higher in some families. But no one knows the reason. Meniere's is said to be "familial" with 7% to 10% of people diagnosed.

Q: Who first discovered Meniere's disease?

A: Prosper Meniere, a French physician, born in Angers, France, in 1799. He was the first to identify a medical condition combining vertigo, hearing loss, and tinnitus, that is now known as Meniere's disease. He finished his medical studies in Paris in 1826 and was hired as a physician-in-chief at the Institute for Deaf and Mute. While working there, he became interested in diseases of the ear.

Q: What year was Meniere's disease accepted?

A: Prosper Meniere formulated a paper on a particular kind of hearing loss and episodic vertigo resulting from lesions of the inner ear in 1861. However, the condition was not medically accepted until the late 19th century. Over 150 years later, the medical profession is still trying to find the cause and cure for Meniere's disease. To date, Meniere's has proven to be an elusive condition to cure.

Q: How is Meniere disease spelled?

A: Two ways. Prosper Meniere was known to write his name as Menière, while his son used the spelling Ménière. Although it is spelled both ways, many people omit the accent marks when writing the word.

Q: What is the definition of Meniere's disease?

A: Meniere's, by definition, is a disorder or disease of the inner ear labyrinth, marked by "unprovoked, recurring, and sudden episodes of disabling vertigo." These episodes are known as 'attacks' that have a fluctuating hearing loss (in the low frequencies) and a sensation of rotational spinning (vertigo), which gives a false sense of movement. The spinning sensation is worse than dizziness. During an 'attack', nausea, vomiting, sweating, tinnitus (ringing and noise in the ears), and a feeling of pressure in the ear often occur. Recurring attacks lead to a permanent hearing loss in the affected ear, and chronic tinnitus.

Q: What is Meniere's disease also known as?

A: Meniere's disease is also known as idiopathic endolymphatic hydrops: Idiopathic referring to a condition of increased hydraulic pressure within the inner ear.

Q: Is there any known cure for Meniere's disease?

A: Unfortunately, there is no known cure for Meniere's disease, no known drug, and no surgical procedure. People who are involved with Meniere's have been searching for the answers since it was discovered and accepted as a medical condition.

Q: Does no known cure mean you can never get better?

A: No cure means there are no medicines, drugs or specific treatments to cure the condition, but that doesn't mean there isn't any way to get better. While there is no specific cure for Meniere's, there are prescribed drugs. These can help control vertigo and cut down the vertigo attacks which are the main problem with this disease.

Q: How long since you recovered from Meniere's?

A: At the time of writing it has been 18 years.

Q: How important was it to be proactive for a recovery?

A: There is growing evidence to suggest that prompt treatment can help prevent the progression of a more chronic long-term course. In my own case, I started a recovery program within the first 3 months. I consider it a major factor in my recovery.

Q: Is Meniere's disease the same as Meniere's syndrome?

A: No. Meniere's disease is of unknown origin or cause, whereas Meniere's syndrome (also known as endolymphatic hydrops) is caused by a specific condition. Meniere's syndrome can occur due to various processes interfering with the normal production and absorption of endolymph e.g. endocrine abnormalities, trauma, electrolyte imbalance, autoimmune diseases, lupus, rheumatoid arthritis, thyroid antibodies, infection, metabolic disturbances, hormonal imbalance, medications, parasitic infections, allergens, hyperlipidemia, and food allergies. If a cause is identified, then you are diagnosed with Meniere's syndrome, not Meniere's disease.

Q: *What is the Meniere's triad?*

A: *The clinical triad in Meniere's consists of three main symptoms: vertigo, tinnitus, and hearing loss.*

Q: *Is Meniere's disease contagious?*

A: *Meniere's disease is not contagious. You can't catch Meniere's like a cold or flu. You can't give Meniere's to another person by contact, using the same utensils or breathing or coughing on them. In a household where one person has Meniere's, there is no chance other family members will be infected or come down with Meniere's; it is simply not infectious.*

Q: *Name five famous people who had Meniere's?*

A: *Famous people who had (or are believed to have had) Meniere's include: Alan Shepard, Vincent Van Gogh, Jonathan Swift, Marilyn Munroe, Marnie Eisenhower,*

Goya, Charles Darwin, Peggy Lee, Martin Luther, Emily Dickinson. The list goes on. There are millions of people with Meniere's alive in the world today.

Q: *How common is Meniere's disease?*

A: *Meniere's is classed as a rare disorder. At the time of writing, it is estimated in the United States, there are 165,000 sufferers and 45,000 new cases diagnosed every year. In the UK, it's estimated that 157 per 100,000 people have Meniere's disease.*

Q: *What is the common age to get Meniere's disease?*

A: *The peak age for Meniere's disease is in the 40-60 year age group.*

Q: *Were you in this age group?*

A: *Yes. I was forty-six years old when I was diagnosed with Meniere's disease.*

Q: *Do both young and old people get Meniere disease?*

A: *Yes. Meniere's disease can be found in almost all ages. It appears in children as young as four and elderly people over the age of 90 years. However, the most common treatment groups range from 49-67 years of age.*

Q: *Is Meniere's more common in Men, or woman?*

A: Both sexes are equally affected although some recent studies show Meniere's disease is slightly more common in women than men.

Q: How can you prevent Meniere's disease?

A: Symptoms develop with no identifiable cause. Without a known cause, there is no known prevention of Meniere's disease.

Q: Are there known risk factors for getting Meniere's?

A: Research is ongoing to find risk factors for Meniere's disease. Factors that can increase risk including a family history and a chemical imbalance in the fluid of the inner ear. There is also evidence that suggests an autoimmune response may be a risk factor, as well as viral infections, and the prevalence of migraines.

Q: Do you have Meniere's in your family?

A: No, not in recent family history, as far as I know.

Q: Can you pass on Meniere's disease to your children?

A: No. However, I did enquire and was assured this was highly unlikely. One of my now adult-children, who was witness to my struggle with Meniere's, is now cautious about the possibility of Meniere's happening in her own life. She has taken the decision to work four days a week to balance between her business and private life. My eldest child is the complete opposite, and a workaholic, just like his dad was. I do worry about him sometimes!

Q: *Did Beethoven have Meniere's disease?*

A: *It is thought so. The musical genius is believed to have suffered from both Meniere's disease and lead poisoning. Beethoven endured hearing loss and eventually went completely deaf. He also suffered from severe tinnitus. He had "harsh roaring" in his ears. Beethoven often complained: "My ears whistle and buzz all day and all night. I can say I am living a wretched life."*

Q: *Is there a difference between dizziness and Meniere's?*

A: *Dizziness is a term used to describe the physical sensation of feeling dizzy, faint or lightheaded. This dizziness can cause you to be unsteady on your feet, stagger, or fall about. Whereas the dizziness experienced with Meniere's disease is rotational vertigo with a sensation of the room spinning around you.*

Q: *What is the difference between vertigo and Meniere's?*

A: *Vertigo is a sensation of an individual's surroundings moving and spinning. Meniere's vertigo is rotational spinning, as if your body is in a vortex.*

Q: *Can you have Meniere's disease without vertigo?*

A: No. To be diagnosed with Meniere's, one must experience uncontrolled episodic rotational vertigo as one of the four Meniere symptoms.

Q: Is labyrinthitis the same as Meniere disease?

A: No. Having suffered from both, the symptoms can be quite similar, but they are two different conditions. Labyrinthitis is an inflammation of the inner ear that can cause episodes of dizziness, nausea, vomiting, eye nystagmus, possible hearing loss, and ringing in the ears. It is also known as vestibular neuritis, caused by a virus, bacterial infection, stress, allergy, reaction to medication or a head injury. I had labyrinthitis after an illness. The symptoms lasted six weeks before suddenly stopping altogether, whereas Meniere's went on for years.

Q: What causes Meniere's disease?

A: Meniere's disease is constantly being re-evaluated. To date, no one knows precisely what causes it. Still, it is believed to result from increased production of inner ear fluid, or a decrease in the re-absorption resulting in excess fluid building up. Why this happens is not exactly known. There have been many theories over the decades.

Q: Can stress cause Meniere's disease?

A: Life stresses, such as the death of close relatives,

is prevalent in a large number of people diagnosed with Meniere disease. But stress has not been identified as a cause for Meniere's disease.

Q: Can migraines cause Meniere's disease?

A: There is a growing body of evidence that Meniere disease and migraine headaches may be related and/or different spectrums of the same disease. Migraines are thought to damage the inner ear, but there is no conclusive research that migraines are the cause of Meniere's disease.

Q: Is Meniere's disease caused by loud music?

A: Exposure to loud music can cause or aggravate tinnitus (ringing in the ears), and cause temporary or permanent hearing loss. Loud music can cause trauma to the sensitive hearing mechanisms, and consequent damage to the ear. However, there is no conclusive evidence that loud noise is an actual cause of Meniere's disease.

Q: Can Meniere's disease be caused by a fall?

A: The causes of Meniere's disease is unknown. Still, in my personal experience, I suffered from a series of traumas to the side of my head, the same side I later experienced unilateral Meniere's. I always wondered about that.

Q: Can a head injury cause Meniere's?

A: Millions of dollars and years of research have been investigating the causes: one of which is the possibility arising from physical trauma, as in head injuries.

Q: Can the herpes virus cause Meniere disease?

A: Some studies have found a find a possible connection with the herpes simplex virus (HSV) but do not conclude that (HSV) causes Meniere's disease. But more studies are needed to determine whether HSV has any effect on the symptoms of Meniere's disease.

Q: Is there a connection between TMJ and Meniere's?

A: There have been reported cases of Meniere's syndrome being relieved through neuromuscular treatment to align the jaw properly. This, in turn, relieved stress on the socket of the TM Joint, and allowed the balance organs, which are extremely close to the socket, to go back to normal as well.

Q: Is Meniere's disease an autoimmune disease?

A: The immune response research for Meniere's disease is focused on inner ear antigens. Approximately one-third of Meniere's disease cases seem to be of an autoimmune origin, although the immunological mechanisms involved are not fully understood.

Q: Do the kidneys have a role to play in Meniere's?

A: *The kidneys and associated hormones produced by unhealthy kidney function are thought to be involved in Meniere's onset. Drinking too much alcohol, eating greasy, sweet, spicy food, or processed food, all affect the kidneys adversely.*

Q: Did Van Gogh, the Impressionist artist, have Meniere's disease?

A: *Art-loving audiologists debate whether it was Meniere's that drove the artist to take his ear, or did the artist Gauguin cut off Van Gogh's earlobe during a fight in a bordello? No one will know for sure, as accounts on events differ through the decades. But from all historical records, the famous Impressionist artist did suffer from a hearing impairment, disabling vertigo, and tinnitus. In his letters, he described classic Meniere symptoms, ringing and roaring in his ears, and intolerance for loud noises.*

Q: Does Meniere's affect the middle ear?

A: *No, it doesn't. It affects the inner ear.*

Q: How does Meniere's affect the inner ear?

A: *When you have Meniere's, fluid builds up in the endolymphatic sac until the membrane that separates the chambers ruptures and floods the nerve of balance, creating a Meniere vertigo attack. Each time you have an attack, the* small cilia in the inner ear are damaged, which results in a progressive hearing loss. Eventually, the affected ear is left with a degree of permanent hearing loss and tinnitus.

Q: What does fluid in the inner ear do?

A: The healthy function of fluids normally present in the inner ear, plays an important role in balance.

Q: What is a healthy inner ear?

A: The inner ear is a group of connected passages known as the labyrinth. The soft structure of the membrane is called the membranous labyrinth. The fluid is held in a membranous structure called the endolymphatic sac. In a normal healthy ear, fluids in the endolymphatic sac are constantly being secreted and reabsorbed. Fluid is maintained at a constant level.

Q: What is unilateral Meniere disease?

A: Unilateral is the term where Meniere's affects one ear. The majority of Meniere's patients are unilateral.

Q: Was your Meniere's unilateral?

A: Yes, only in my right ear.

Q: Can you get Meniere's in the other ear?

A: Some sufferers are bilateral, (Meniere's in both ears), or become bilateral at a later date.

Q: What's the risk of getting Meniere's in both ears?

A: The risk of developing the disease in the opposite ear is, unfortunately, estimated to be as high as thirty percent.

Q: When is bilateral Meniere's likely to happen?

A: Most doctors believe that if you are going to suffer bilateral Meniere's, the symptoms will usually occur in the unaffected ear within two to five years from the onset of Meniere's in the first ear.

Q: What are episodic Meniere's disease symptoms?

A: Episodic symptoms are aural fullness, tinnitus, and disabling rotational vertigo. As the word indicates, they can appear unprovoked at any time.

Q: What are fluctuating symptoms?

A: When symptoms fluctuate, they vary in intensity and duration. During an attack, hearing loss may fluctuate. Vertigo severity may be more or less. After the attack, your hearing loss may be severe but it will return to normal levels a few hours later. Tinnitus may be louder before, during, or after an attack. Most every episode is unpredictable, which makes no one attack the same. Symptoms can be more intense or less than the previous attack.

Q: *What triggered your Meniere's symptoms?*

A: *Mental, emotional, and physical stress have been identified as triggers. Stress, emotional distress, overwork, fatigue, visual disturbances, excessive tiredness from extended activities, pressure changes, excessive salt, food allergies, and illness, can set off attacks.*

Q: *What famous people today have Meniere's?*

A: *Famous people today who have (or are thought to have) Meniere's are David Alstead - pianist, Steve Francis - professional basketball player - Dana Davis - author, Mike Reilly - American League, Ryan Adams, Katie Le Clerc - television and movie actor, Andrew Knight - editor, journalist, and media baron, the late Les Paul - jazz guitarist, Jessica Williams - American pianist and composer, Kristen Chenoweth - American singer, musical theatre, film and television actress and author. Meniere's is not selective about who suffers it.*

Q: *What is the Tullio phenomenon ?*

A: *Tullio phenomenon happens when a change in pressure sets off dizziness, nausea, and nystagmus. Nose-blowing, swallowing, straining to lift heavy objects, loud music, or even the sound of your voice can set off vertigo, imbalance,* and eye movement, hearing loss and tinnitus. Meniere's syndrome is the most common cause of the Tullio phenomenon.

Q: *Is Meniere's a debilitating disease?*

A: *Attacks of Meniere's are incredibly debilitating. At the time of rotational vertigo, you can't do anything but lay down. The spinning sensation can be violent. Accompanying nausea, vomiting, sweating, and imbalance are all overwhelming and out of control. So yes, the symptoms are debilitating.*

Q: *Is Meniere's a serious disease?*

A: *Meniere's disease is serious in its physical and mental effects, creating anxiety, depression, stress, tinnitus, and hearing loss. However, it is not a terminal disease.*

Q: *Is Meniere's a chronic condition?*

A: *Yes, it can be. If the sufferer is experiencing the symptoms of intermittent, unpredictable and frequent attacks of debilitating vertigo, loss of balance, nausea, vomiting, dizziness, as well as varying degrees of symptoms such as hearing loss, mild vertigo with dizziness, mild or severe tinnitus, and sensitivity to sound over a long period, it is chronic. Symptoms vary from person to another. One sufferer's symptoms will not be the same as another, although sufferers will experience all the symptoms at some stage.*

Q: *Can you die from Meniere's?*

A: *This question is the one I am asked most often. Although you might wish for a place in heaven, during the darkest days of vertigo attacks, Meniere's is not terminal, and you won't die from it.*

Q: *Is Meniere's a progressive disease?*

A: *Meniere's is known to be a progressive disease with three stages.*

Q: *Are the stages of Meniere's the same for everyone?*

A: *Not at all, the stages vary in individuals.*

Q: *What is stage one of Meniere's?*

A: *Stage one is the early Meniere's onset. This is marked by unpredictable attacks of vertigo that happen without any warning. Other symptoms in stage one are fluctuating hearing loss, a fullness in the ear, and tinnitus.*

Q: *Does Tinnitus precede an attack in stage one?*

A: *Often this is the case.*

Q: *What happens to your hearing between attacks?*

A: *In the first stage, between attacks, the hearing returns to normal.*

Q: *What is the usual period between attacks?*

A: *The period between attacks can be hours, days, or weeks. It varies from person to person.*

Q: *What is stage two of Meniere's?*

A: *In stage two, vertigo attacks continue, along with increased tinnitus and fluctuating hearing loss.*

Q: *In stage two, do you have warnings of an attack?*

A: *Yes. Tinnitus increases before an attack, as well as 'wooziness' and aural fullness.*

Q: *What happens to your hearing in stage two?*

A: *Hearing continues to fluctuate after vertigo attacks. Unfortunately, each attack brings about progressive, permanent hearing loss.*

Q: *Is Tinnitus worse during stage two?*

A: *Yes. Tinnitus gets worse. Tinnitus becomes more intrusive and demanding.*

Q: *What is stage three of Meniere's?*

A: *Stage three is the late stage of Meniere's. Attacks of vertigo get less frequent, may not last as long, and are often less violent.*

Q: *What happens to your hearing in stage three?*

A: *Hearing loss can be severe in the affected ear. Loud noises can cause problems. Your hearing is still fluctuating at this stage, so a hearing device, from my experience, is impossible to program because of this. Permanent and hearing loss and continual tinnitus can be the cause of depression.*

Q: *How long does Meniere's disease last?*

A: *Meniere's may persist for 30 years or more. Vertigo attacks can persist for decades, although with a gradual decline after ten years.*

Q: *Can Meniere's go into remission?*

A: *Meniere's is an unpredictable illness. Meniere's disease is different for each patient. You can experience temporary spontaneous remissions between attacks, from hours, days, weeks, months, or sometimes several years when Meniere's is active. Between attacks, you can continue to have a sense of wooziness and a feeling of instability.*

Q: *Can Meniere's burn out?*

A: *Yes. After a number of years, vertigo attacks may be less frequent and reduce in intensity. Hearing loss will stabilize at a moderate to severe level. This is called burning out, but unfortunately, this is not the case for everyone.*

Q: *Does burning-out mean Meniere's has gone?*

A: *Unfortunately not. It means two things: hearing in the affected ear has been permanently destroyed; attacks have reduced in intensity or have stopped altogether. But, Meniere's can still show as active.*

Q: *When can I expect Meniere's disease to go away?*

A: *You will find no one can answer that. For me, Meniere's did go away. I also experienced a significant relief in the intensity and frequency of attacks well before I made a full recovery. The faded bell curve on the audiogram shows I once had Meniere's, but now Meniere's is something I had in my past medical history.*

Q: *Is every person's Meniere's experience the same?*

A: *No. Your experience will be different from my own because Meniere's disease affects people differently. My experience was frequent acute (severe) rotational vertigo attacks. In contrast, other sufferers I talked to, experienced acute vertigo attacks, but less frequently. Others reported less severe attacks, and they were able to continue working, (and surf the internet), whereas other people are forced to give up work. Many sufferers are unable to use the computer.*

Q: *Is Meniere's disease curable?*

A: *No, it's not curable. While there is no one known cure for Meniere's, Meniere's can undoubtedly go away. I recovered by managing symptoms and allowing my body to heal; a healthy body is not a place for a disease.*

Q: Were you lucky to have recovered from Meniere's?

A: I don't see the recovery I made as lucky. The prognosis was for a disease for a lifetime, which I never personally accepted. I don't think recovery is about luck at all. For me, it was a determination to get better.

Q: How bad can Meniere's disease get?

A: Do I have to answer that one? I had very bad days where I wouldn't have wished Meniere's on my worst enemy. Intolerable! I worked out what might be exasperating the symptoms and took those aspects out of my life. The more I understood what was happening during attacks, I more I believed Meniere's symptoms could be managed effectively. I can't stress enough how much you can manage symptoms, and get better from this otherwise debilitating disease.

Q: Are there complications from Meniere's disease?

A: While Meniere's disease doesn't cause physical complications as such, it makes life distressing, challenging, and complicated. The symptoms cause fear, lack of confidence, unreliability, and emotional stress. This can lead to anger, depression, and other psychological problems, which often need professional help. The permanent hearing loss in the affected ear is a complication of Meniere's. However, once your hearing has stabilized, the loss can be overcome with hearing devices. Another complication from Meniere's is balance issues leading to accidents like falls in the home.

Q: *Did you take a fall due to balance issues?*

A: *Yes, once. I slipped from the top rung of a ladder, dropping the five liter can of paint I was holding. The white paint emptied over the newly polished timber floor. Guess who had to clean up!*

Q: *What is your life expectancy with Meniere's?*

A: *Life expectancy is the same as if you didn't have Meniere's disease.*

Q: *Is your quality of life affected by Meniere's?*

A: *The research quantifies that Meniere sufferers lose 43.9% from the optimum wellbeing position of normal people. In acute episodes, the wellbeing scale is recorded by sufferers, as being at the same level found in patients facing terminal diseases, such as cancer.*

Q: *What is The Quality of Wellbeing Scale?*

A: *The Quality of Wellbeing Scale is a recognized*

scientific study applied to many aspects of human life. In the study, Meniere sufferers are the most severely impaired non-hospitalized patients studied so far. Meniere's (when people with Meniere's were not having acute episodes) is comparable to very ill adults with a life-threatening illness, such as Cancer or Aids. The Quality of Wellbeing for Meniere's sufferers, when having acute attacks, is closer to an Aids victim, or a Cancer patient —six days before death.

Q: *What is the DHI?*

A: *The Jacobson's Dizziness Handicap Inventory (DHI) is a subjective test that helps a sufferer to explain the impact vertigo is having on their life. It consists of 25 questions about vertigo, which measure the degree of physical, emotional, and functional disability.*

Q: *What are the long-term physical effects of Meniere's?*

A: *The physical side effects are moderate to severe hearing loss, and chronic tinnitus.*

Q: *What are the long-term emotional effects?*

A: *As well as having a physical effect, I would say Meniere's is also a psychological trauma that affects your sense of wellbeing. One of the primary psychological effects is the loss of confidence socially. There is also a prevailing loss of confidence in the immediate future.*

Q: Does Meniere's disease make you stupid?

A: No, not that I have noticed, or been told so far!

Q: Can Meniere's cause cognitive issues?

A: Yes. Cognitive issues persist while Meniere's is active. Research has shown Meniere sufferers show a decreased ability to multi-task without confusion, have trouble keeping track of the relevant subject in conversation, show a marked decrease in mental stamina, have difficulty grasping whole concepts, and difficulty with memory recall. Over the longterm there is no decline in mental ability.

Q: What makes Meniere's disease symptoms flare up?

A: No one knows for sure, but there are now numerous, well-documented known 'triggers' that can exasperate symptoms, from dietary triggers like too much salt to physical triggers like stress. Keeping a personal diary of attacks and possible causes of the attack (triggers) helps clarify what aggravates symptoms. The more aware you are of possible causes, the more you can avoid attacks and the more control you have over Meniere's and the less out of control the disease makes you feel.

Q: Can kidney function affect Meniere's symptoms?

A: According to traditional Oriental medicine the kidneys influence the ears and hearing. If your kidneys are weak, then the normal functioning of the ears will be affected. Also, the kidneys can only be nourished by the right nutrition. So you can stabilize the kidneys by eating well. A strong function of the kidney system will help the deficiency that shows up as dizziness and tinnitus.

Q: Why is smoking bad for Meniere's?

A: Smoking restricts blood vessels, which in turn affects blood circulation in the inner ear. Limited blood supply to anywhere in your body means that the part of your body that needs the healing substances carried in your blood will suffer i.e., your ear. Your body is constantly replacing itself on a cellular level, so make sure you take the opportunity to make yourself stronger and better than ever before. Make sure your body gets as much healthy blood as possible.

Q: Is passive smoke bad for Meniere's?

A: Yes. Don't accept second-hand smoke. It's a health hazard that does you absolutely no good. Breathe in someone else's exhalation, and you take poisons and toxic chemicals into your own body. This is to say environmental pollution doesn't help Meniere's symptoms.

Q: Does Meniere's disease cause fatigue?

A: Yes. As the balance organ in the inner ear/ears is damaged, the brain, the eyes, muscles, and entire balance system are compensating, second by second,. This is why you feel so tired. Physical, emotional, and mental fatigue are triggers for attacks, so tiredness and fatigue are something you have to manage.

Q: Did Meniere's make you tired?

A: Meniere's certainly made me dog-tired most of the time. I often looked pale, drained of life, thoroughly washed out, and had virtually no energy. I worried my family with that exhausted look; as initially, it was a constant state of my being.

Q: What did you do when you felt tired?

A: Tiredness was not a good state to be in. So I made sure I took heed of how I was feeling. Whenever I felt tired, regardless of what I was doing, I stopped and took a nap, or meditated. If I pushed anything when I was tired, inevitably, I would have an attack.

Q: What practical things did you do to combat fatigue?

A: I stopped stacking one thing on top of another, which was my habit. I learned that it was OK to leave a full in-tray, that things could wait, and nothing was stamped urgent. I had to stop trying to do everything in a short space of time but to spread the load and responsibilities. Once I did that, I noticed a significant reduction in attacks.

Q: *What advice do you have to manage fatigue?*

A: *Counter the tiredness by consistently practicing relaxation. Take time out for yourself. Pace yourself, taking care not to get over-tired; over-worked, or over-extend yourself during activities.*

Q: *Are frequent headaches common with Meniere's disease?*

A: *If you are prone to headaches and migraines, and you have Meniere's disease, you are more likely to suffer from severe headaches or migraines with vertigo attacks. Headaches do follow attacks and often appear due to fatigue.*

Q: *Do you get headaches with Meniere's?*

A: *Up to my diagnosis I never rarely had a headache unless it was the hangover kind. During Meniere's, I went through headache medication like candy some days.*

Q: *Did sinus or colds affect your Meniere's symptoms?*

A: *No. I didn't get sinus infections or suffer unduly with colds. Flu aggravated symptoms of tiredness and wooziness, it did seem to increase the feeling of instability. During the flu season, I made an effort to avoid colds or flu with hand washing, avoiding contact with sick people, and taking extra vitamins. I would also take my vitamin and supplement booster regime at the change of seasons.*

Q: *Do barometric pressure and weather affect Meniere's symptoms?*

A: *Yes. It is well documented that Meniere's patients are sensitive to changes in weather. The diseased fluid-filled inner ear is very sensitive to barometric pressure changes. For this reason, spring and fall are notably 'bad seasons' for sufferers. I correlated barometric pressure with the onset of my attacks or at least during the first stage.*

Q: *Did you ever feel lightheaded?*

A: *I call it woozy. Yes, most of the time.*

Q: *Does Meniere's cause memory loss?*

A: *Cognitive research shows that Meniere's can decrease your ability to retrieve memories.*

Q: *Is Meniere's disease brain fog real?*

A: *Brain fog is not a medical symptom used in diagnosing Meniere's disease. Brain fog is described as forgetting things, having trouble remembering, feeling disoriented, and confused. These symptoms are common when you suffer from a chronic medical condition. I experienced constant brain fog to different degrees in the early stages of Meniere's but not since I've recovered.*

Q: *Can Meniere's disease cause seizures?*

A: Meniere's disease doesn't cause seizures, but if you are prone to seizures, the physiological effects of having Meniere's may exasperate seizure symptoms.

Q: Does Meniere's disease cause blackouts?

A: No, Meniere's doesn't cause blackouts.

Q: Can Meniere's disease cause a loss of consciousness?

A: No. Meniere's would only cause loss of consciousness is if you lost your balance, fell, banged your head, and knocked yourself out.

Q: Can Meniere's disease cause a stiff neck?

A: No, Meniere's doesn't cause a stiff neck. However, periods of acute vertigo with nystagmus, plus the head tension of constant balance correction can give you a stiff neck.

Q: Does Meniere's disease cause itchy ears?

A: No, Meniere's doesn't cause itchy ears. It does cause aural fullness.

Q: Does Meniere's disease cause jaw pain?

A: No. Meniere's does not cause jaw pain.

Q: Does Meniere's disease cause joint pain?

A: No. Meniere's doesn't cause joint pain.

Q: Can Meniere's disease cause abdominal pain?

A: Meniere's is known to cause diarrhea and associated abdominal irritation during a vertigo attack.

Q: Does Meniere's disease cause excessive sweating?

A: Cold sweats are the result of vertigo. In the middle of an attack, you can break out in a cold sweat. Tension over threatening Meniere situations, such as constant loud noise or visual disturbances, can cause one to sweat.

Q: Does blood pressure affect Meniere's disease?

A: Blood pressure can increase during a vertigo attack, but blood pressure doesn't affect Meniere's disease.

Q: Did Meniere's give you high blood pressure?

A: No, not at all.

Q: Can Meniere's cause heart palpitations?

A: Meniere's vertigo attack brings fear, stress, and anxiety in its wake. Depending on how your body's fight-flight reflex kicks in, heart palpitations are possible.

Q: Can Meniere's effect sleep?

A: Yes. Meniere's affects sleep patterns. If you sleep for long periods during the day, you have less of a good night's sleep. If you are tired, you are more prone to an attack, so it can be a vicious circle to manage and cope.

Q: Can Meniere's make you depressed?

A: Yes, it sure can. Changes in mood are common, and for a good reason. Meniere's brings a lot of complications, discomfort, and loss of wellbeing. Some people find they need to take a course of prescribed antidepressants or anti-anxiety medication or seek counsel with a health professional.

Q: What did you do about depression?

A: I didn't ignore feelings of depression. On 'dark days,' I talked to a professional about how Meniere's was making me feel. This helped me work through issues.

Q: What are other mood changes that can happen?

A: Anger, irritability, fear, anxiety, impatience, and a lack of confidence.

Q: What brought out your pessimistic side?

A: Two things; I couldn't socialize effectively, and an overwhelming fear of non-recovery.

ON THE QUESTION OF DIAGNOSIS

Q: Who diagnoses Meniere's disease?

A: You can't self-diagnose Meniere's disease. Only a registered medical professional, a General Practitioner, ENT Specialist, or Meniere's disease specialist can prescribe a series of tests to conclude a diagnosis of Meniere's disease and advise you with treatment.

Q: Is Meniere's disease easy to diagnose?

A: Yes, a diagnosis of Meniere's disease requires two episodes of vertigo, each lasting 20 minutes or longer (but not longer than 24 hours) and a specific range of hearing loss, verified by a hearing test.

Q: How is Meniere's diagnosed?

A: The doctor will ask you to describe your symptoms

and what happens during an attack. The doctor will order tests: blood tests, hearing tests, an MRI or CT scan, other tests to check your balance and neurological tests to rule out any brain issues.

Q: *Does Meniere's show on an MRI?*

A: *Meniere's doesn't show on an MRI. Other diseases that have similar symptoms, such as a vestibular migraine, viral labyrinthitis, or a brainstem stroke, will show up. The gadolinium-enhanced MRI checks the interior auditory canals, and this helps to rule out other causes.*

Q: *Can you see Meniere's disease on an MRI scan?*

A: *The MRI scan uses a strong magnetic field, not x-rays. MRI scans will not show which ear is affected or how severe the Meniere's is, or confirm a diagnosis of Meniere's disease. The scan can show the internal auditory canal and exclude brain tumors and multiple sclerosis. The MRI scan is a diagnosis of exclusion. This is probably the most important and reassuring element of the MRI scan.*

Q: *Is there a test for Meniere's disease?*

A: *There is no definitive test for Meniere's disease. However, there are two tests specific for Meniere's disease: the glycerol dehydration test, which involves ingesting a dehydrating agent called glycerol, and observing two things;*

a change in symptoms and a measurable improvement in hearing. The second specific test is electrocochleography (ECoG). In this test, electrical information received from the inner ear is recorded and compared. In people with Meniere's disease, the information is significantly different than other conditions of the ear.

Q: *Is there a blood test for Meniere's disease?*

A: *There is no specific blood test that indicates Meniere's disease. A blood test workup when you present with Meniere's symptoms can help eliminate other possible issues, such as infection present in the body.*

Q: *Why are so many different tests used in the diagnosis of Meniere's?*

A: *Meniere's is not defined by its symptoms. There are many disorders that have the same symptoms as Meniere's disease, so a series of diagnostic tests are needed to eliminate other conditions. Migraines and ear infections, which is also known to affect balance and hearing, can have the same disturbing symptoms.*

Q: *How is a correct diagnosis made?*

A: *A qualified medical professional makes a diagnosis by excluding other diseases with similar symptoms. If a cause for symptoms is found, then, by definition, the diagnosis will* not be Meniere's disease, but some other condition. If you have the same Meniere symptoms, but no cause is found, then the diagnosis will be Meniere's disease.

Q: *How is an audiogram used in diagnosis?*

A: *Meniere's is diagnosed by a hearing test called an audiogram. An audiogram performed by a technician is a non-invasive, painless hearing test. The hearing is tested in each ear through headphones. An audiometer delivers sounds of specific frequencies (pure tones) at different intensities to determine how loud a sound must be, to be perceived for each frequency. The results are compared to the normal hearing on each frequency on a computer graph. In Meniere's, the results show a low-frequency sensorineural hearing loss in the affected ear that fluctuates between tests.*

Q: *What are the Weber test and the Rinne tests?*

A: *These non-invasive, painless tests use a metal tuning fork to differentiate conductive from sensorineural hearing loss. Hearing loss in Meniere's disease is a sensorineural hearing loss. Sensorineural hearing loss (SNHL) is a type of hearing loss, or deafness, in which the root cause lies in the inner ear or sensory organ (cochlea and associated structures), or the vestibulocochlear nerve (cranial nerve VIII), or neural part.*

Q: *What happens in a Rinne test?*

A: A hearing by bone and air conduction test where the stem of a vibrating tuning fork is held against the mastoid bone, the bone behind the ear (bone conduction of sound); as soon as the sound is no longer perceived, the tuning fork is taken away and held close to the ear (air conduction). In normal hearing, the fork can still be heard, which indicates that the air conduction is better than bone conduction. With conductive hearing loss, bone conduction is louder than air conduction. With sensorineural hearing loss, both air and bone conduction are reduced, but air conduction is louder at testing.

Q: What happens in the Weber test?

A: This is used to test unilateral sensorineural hearing loss. A tuning fork is placed on the midline of the head, and you indicate in which ear the tone is louder. In the unilateral sensorineural hearing loss, the tone is louder in the normal ear because the tuning fork stimulates both inner ears equally. The patient perceives the sound stimulus louder in the unaffected ear.

Q: What is speech audiometry?

A: A test on speech recognition where you are presented with a list of words with two equally accentuated syllables such as 'staircase', 'baseball', 'bookshelf'; spoken at specific sound intensities, and you repeat them. The Audiologist notes the intensity at which you repeat 50% of the words.

Q: *Are there other hearing tests?*

A: *Yes. Word recognition score tests using one-syllable words to test the ability to discriminate speech sounds; tympanometry which measures the impedance of the middle ear to acoustic energy; acoustic reflex which helps eliminate a tumor on the auditory nerve.*

Q: *Were any of the hearing tests painful?*

A: *No, they were all easy, non-invasive and painless.*

Q: *Did you go to a hospital for the tests?*

A: *No. The ENT specialist gave me a referral to an Audiologist. I made an appointment and went to her office and she had the diagnostic machines there. The tests were thorough but didn't take long.*

Q: *What was the strangest test you had?*

A: *I had a non-invasive test called an auditory brain stem response. I sat with a latex cap on my head, rather like ones used to monitor sleep apnea, and was told to relax while the technician attached numerous surface electrodes with colored wires. These monitored brainwave responses to acoustic stimulation. The resulting brainwave patterns were fed into a computer, to rule out a tumor on the brainstem. Luckily I didn't have one.*

Q: Can you have a mild form of Meniere's disease?

A: Meniere's disease symptoms vary from person to person. No one patient has the same experiences, although the symptoms are the same. Some people I spoke with had a mild onset of symptoms they hardly noticed. Other people, like myself, experienced rapid onset and violent symptoms. Meniere's disease can progress slowly or rapidly and the symptoms can vary from mild to severe. Even day to day symptoms can be severe and on other days, mild.

Q: Can Meniere's be misdiagnosed?

A: Quite possibly. There are diseases, known and unknown, that have the same symptoms as Meniere's disease. Patients could be misdiagnosed with Meniere's and yet be treated for Meniere's. That is why it is important to get a specialist's opinion. While relatively easy to diagnose, medical professionals don't agree on the prognosis and outcome of Meniere's disease. This makes it difficult for the patient to put a successful management plan in place.

ON THE QUESTION OF TREATMENT

Q: Is Meniere's disease considered to be a neurological problem?

A: No, it's not considered to be a neurological problem. Meniere's disease affects the inner ear and balance system, therefore it's considered to be a problem of the ear. An Ear, Nose and Throat (ENT) specialist treats it.

Q: Who is the best doctor for Meniere's disease?

A: In my case, my general practitioner referred me to an Ear Nose and Throat (ENT) specialist who knew about Meniere's disease. The ENT specialist turned out to be the best person for me.

Q: What was the most significant thing your specialist told you?

A: As far as management of Meniere's disease from a patient perspective, there wasn't a lot to tell me at the time, except, he did say to give up salt and walk away from stress. What he said made me wonder what other things I should walk away from and give up.

Q: How is Meniere's disease treated medically?

A: There are many possible treatments for the symptoms of Meniere's disease, from outpatient procedures, vestibular balance training and/or surgery, plus of course medications.

Q: What is gentamicin treatment?

A: The endolymphatic sac is the immune organ of the inner ear. The theory of immune involvement has created a trend towards procedures aimed at destroying the endolymphatic sac. It is reported Meniere attacks stop when the immune system of the ear is destroyed or suppressed. Destroying the endolymph involves an outpatient procedure, where gentamicin is injected into the eardrum. Recently it has been reported one injection has been successful in stopping vertigo. I understand you can expect four of these injections administered over a month and this will stop vertigo for about a year. If the dizziness returns, another series of injections of gentamicin are given.

Q: Were gentamicin injections an option you considered?

A: No. Never. In recent years (intratympanic steroid, gentamycin) have been tried in patients with Meniere's disease. Not all surgeons recommend it as it is still a relatively new procedure and the long-term effectiveness and side effects are not well documented. The use of intratympanic dexamethasone has gained popularity over gentamicin for the treatment of Meniere's disease in recent years.

Q: What is shunt surgery for Meniere's disease?

A: Lymphatic Sac Shunt is an outpatient procedure thought to preserve hearing and relieves vertigo. The probability of needing to repeat the operation is high because the shunt has a tendency to become blocked and needs replacing. The shunt is a procedure rated by some as having no more benefit than doing nothing at all.

Q: Was shunt surgery a procedure you considered?

A: My ENT surgeon did explain the operation to me, but I didn't consider having surgery as part of my management for Meniere's. So much is unknown about the condition, treatments vary depending on the surgeon and each specialist has a preferred method for treating Meniere's. Surgeons are constantly changing views on surgical procedures related to Meniere's. At the time of writing, there appears to be no ultimate surgical answer.

Q: *What is vestibular neurectomy for Meniere's disease?*

A: *Vestibular Neurectomy includes surgically cutting the vestibular nerve (the nerve of balance). Severing the nerve of balance stops that information being sent to the brain.*

Q: *Did you consider vestibular neurectomy?*

A: *Never. Vestibular neurectomy is invasive radical surgery and I was not into that idea at all. I found the idea of invasive surgery frightening. I prefer to take matters into my own hands, to retain control over outcomes. My friend went through this surgery. The procedure resulted in serious problems for him. He still had Meniere's, which went bilateral a year after the surgery.*

Q: *Did you have any surgery or invasive medical procedures?*

A: *I chose to avoid all surgery and invasive procedures. I decided to self-manage the condition instead. For me, this proved to be the right thing to do. But in the end it is a personal choice.*

Q: *What would you say to someone contemplating surgery?*

A: *Regardless of acute symptoms, I'd say, don't rush into what may seem to be an easy or quick solution. If surgery is being offered to you, ask questions about the associated risk,* *prognosis and success rate.*

Q: Should you get a second opinion?

A: Yes, for sure. Get a second and third medical opinion for treatment. I am adamant about this. It is a serious decision for you to consider.

Q: Did you ever think of surgery or procedures as a quick cure?

A: No. Not for me. It comes down to personal health choices. But I have met a number of people who rushed into surgery hoping for a quick 'cure' only to see them years later battling Meniere symptoms again. They were not over Meniere's despite the surgeries and procedures and most were understandably embittered and constantly seeking or waiting for a 'magic cure' or procedure.

Q: If you didn't opt for surgery, what did you do?

A: I took two prescribed medications, and embarked on a holistic approach to getting well which included lifestyle changes, low-salt diet, increased exercise, stress management, natural remedies, and meditation. The holistic management of Meniere's worked well for me. It was not a quick fix, and it didn't happen overnight. But it did work, and now I no longer have Meniere's disease.

Q: What are new treatments for Meniere's disease?

A: The medical profession is constantly trying new procedures in its effort to find treatments. Will the medical profession in the future agree one surgical or medical procedure? Everyone involved in Meniere's is waiting to see.

Q: Can Meniere's disease be treated naturally?

A: At the time of writing, there is no known proven natural cure for Meniere's, just the same as there is no proven medical cure. However, Meniere's disease symptoms can be managed naturally; from vitamins, supplements, meditation, acupuncture, breathing techniques, exercise, stress management, and spending time in nature. Ten years ago, I compiled a personal list of 100 ways to help Meniere symptoms, each one on the list, still just as relevant today.

ON THE QUESTION OF MEDICATION

Q: What medications did you take for Meniere disease?

A: Nost many. I was prescribed three. I took just two on a daily basis: a fluid pressure suppressant (diuretic) and an anti-nausea drug.

Q: Which diuretic did you take for Meniere's disease?

A: My Specialist prescribed Serc (Betahistine dihydrochloride).

Q: How does Serc help Meniere's?

A: It's thought to reduce the pressure in the inner ear, reducing the episodes of Meniere attacks.

Q: Was Betahistine effective for you?

A: Some people question its effectiveness. However, I found that if I missed a dose, I'd experience increased tinnitus and a woozy unstable feeling leading to an attack. Initially, these symptoms were enough to make me stay on this medication until I was better.

Q: What diuretic did you take?

A: I took Kaluri, the brand name for the chemical Amiloride. It increases urinary output which in turn flushes out sodium (salt). Amiloride is prescribed as a preferred diuretic because it retains potassium in the body.

Q: What are the side effects of a non-potassium sparing diuretic?

A: Diuretics can cause a loss of potassium so it is important to take a potassium supplement. Potassium is essential for the proper functioning of the kidneys, heart, nerves and digestive system. Diuretics taken longer than six months can dramatically reduce levels of folic acid in the body. Lack of folic acid creates a toxic amino acid associated with hardening of the arteries. If you suffer from high cholesterol, take a folic acid supplement.

Q: What medications did you take for an acute vertigo attack?

A: For nausea and vomiting, I would take Stemitol,

an anti-nausea drug used in the treatment of acute Meniere attacks. I took a tablet as soon as an attack started in an attempt to minimize the spinning sensation and nausea.

Q: Did you ever need a shot of Stemitol?

A: Yes. Once or twice I was given a shot of Stemitol in a severe attack by my G.P who made a house call. Shots of Stemitol were fast-acting and effective.

Q: Did you ever go to the A & E during an acute vertigo attack?

A: Only during the first vertigo attack. My wife rang the A&E department and explained my symptoms. The A&E advised she take me down, but I was too ill to go anywhere. So she rang the ambulance and a paramedic team turned up. After examining me, they concluded it was a middle ear problem. Following that vertigo attack, I went to a specialist and was I was diagnosed with Meniere's.

Q: Did you take painkillers?

A: I didn't need to take regular painkillers for Meniere's disease symptoms.

Q: Did you take over the counter medicine for Meniere's?

A: No.

Q: Did you try any antiviral medications?

A: No, I didn't take any antiviral medication.

Q: Any other medications such as Meclizine, Orthokine or Klonopin?

A: No, just the three I outlined previously. Drugs can mask the problem and in no way solve it. Meclizine is often prescribed, but this medication only inhibits the central nervous system and inhibits neural transmission to the vestibular system, which could make balance worse.

Q: What is oto-104 for Meniere's disease?

A: Increasing evidence implicating autoimmunity in Meniere's disease, has seen the corticosteroid steroid intratympanic dexamethasone gain in popularity over gentamycin. Being a minor surgical procedure; patients can be discharged on the same day.

Q: Did you take steroids to help treat Meniere's ?

A: Personally speaking I didn't consider steroids as part of symptom management. I was not prepared to be part of any medical trials in that regard. However, corticosteroids, by their anti-inflammatory and immunosuppressive action, are becoming increasingly more popular as a method for controlling vertigo.

Q: Do you take medication now you are well? When did you stop?

A: I don't take any medications, now I have recovered and haven't done so for over 18 years now. When I was symptom-free, my specialist told me I would need to take Serc for the rest of my life. I wasn't happy about that. So once I felt better, after a great deal of thought, I cautiously reduced the Serc dosage down, cutting the tablets into tiny quarters until I was off the drug altogether. Mind you, I don't advocate going against doctor's orders.

ON THE QUESTION OF VERTIGO

Q: What gives us our sense of balance?

A: The balance system is made up of three sources that feed information to the brain: vision (through your eyes you see where you are going); sensors in the body (muscles, joints and feet) to feel how you move and sense where you are moment to moment; the inner ear (vestibular organ) signals the brain when your head, neck or any part of your body moves.

Q: Why does Meniere's disease affect balance?

A: Because Meniere's adversely affects the vestibular system which is one of our main balance mechanisms.

Q: What happens to the balance system in Meniere's?

A: The vestibular system receives sensory information, such as motion, equilibrium, and spatial orientation for the purpose of co-ordinating this information for spatial balance. The vestibular system is also responsible for transmitting this co-ordinated information to the brain. Active Meniere's affects the vestibular system and inhibits balance information being sent to the brain. That is why you end up with a balance issue with Meniere's.

Q: When vertigo symptoms occur, what is it called?

A: It is called an 'attack'.

Q: Do you get warnings prior to Meniere's vertigo attacks?

A: Yes. Any of the following symptoms often indicated the beginning stage of a vertigo attack: Increased tinnitus/ loud roaring, aural fullness, increased tiredness/yawning for no apparent reason, feeling off-balance and decreased hearing. This means the Reissner membrane is already being stretched by fluid build up in one of the endolymphatic sacs. These symptoms can happen over a day or two or within half an hour.

Q: Did symptoms always warn you of an impending vertigo attack?

A: Yes. I learned to pay attention to symptoms and to

take action immediately. *Warning symptoms became essential warning tools for managing my attacks.*

Q: *Can you describe a typical warning of an attack?*

A: *There was often an 'aura' where some (or all) of the following specific symptoms warned me of an oncoming vertigo attack. Prior to an attack, I would feel less stable, experiencing a slight loss of balance, along with a woozy feeling or lightheadedness. Sometimes I would get a crashing headache. I always noticed a sensation of increased pressure in the ear, as if my ear was stuffed with cotton wool. External sounds became more muffled. As tinnitus increased, hearing decreased.*

Q: *Why is it important to recognize symptoms of a vertigo attack?*

A: *The sooner you recognize this beginning stage the better. If you take action, you have more opportunity of avoiding the attack or lessening the intensity. Whatever you do, take this beginning stage seriously. If you are experiencing the beginning symptoms of a Meniere's vertigo attack, you need to put measures in place immediately. Don't ignore them. This may mean resting mentally and physically for a day.*

Q: *Are nausea and vomiting symptoms of Meniere's?*

A: *No, nausea and vomiting are symptoms of many*

diseases, but not actual symptoms of Meniere's disease; rather they are caused by rotational vertigo, which is a Meniere symptom. Feeling queasy, nauseous, sick to your stomach and vomiting are symptoms felt during vertigo attacks.

Q: *What happens during a Meniere's vertigo attack?*

A: *In the beginning, you experience serious dizziness which is quickly developing into nystagmus, where your eyes feel like they're following the room moving around you. This may take place over three to four minutes, but you are still mobile enough to find a place to lie down. After that, you are into an acute rotational spinning vertigo attack. This lasts for at least thirty minutes to an hour.*

Q: *How did you cope with Meniere's vertigo attacks?*

A: *First, I understood what was happening during attacks. This was very important. Then I figured out the pattern of attacks. This put me more in control of the attack at any point. I learned to recognize the beginning, middle, and end stages of attacks. Then I figured out what I could do at every stage to help myself cope and manage. This helped the attacks get less violent and less frequent until I no longer had attacks at all.*

Q: *How does the Meniere attack finish?*

A: *Towards the end of the attack you will notice the*

spinning is a little less severe. As the spinning slows down, you are managing to see something specific in the room, before it spins away. Slowly you are able to focus on a spot or a picture. Once focusing on an object becomes possible, you start feeling you can get control back. Finally, there is no more spinning and you may be able to sleep.

Q: *Is the intensity of vertigo attacks always the same?*

A: *No. The intensity at one end can be mild: feeling woozy, lightheaded and a little unstable. At the other end of the scale, one is caught up in a spinning nightmare.*

Q: *How often do attacks happen?*

A: *Attacks vary in frequency. They can happen as much as one every three days. I've had what I describe as cluster attacks. These happen every few days and go on like this for two or three weeks.*

Q: *How long does an attack last?*

A: *Meniere's disease symptoms come on as 'episodes' or 'attacks.' Attacks vary in frequency and intensity. Attacks can last from 20 minutes to one hour.*

Q: *Can one attack be followed by another?*

A: *Unfortunately, yes. You can have weeks, where one attack, is followed by another.*

Q: *Did you have days when you felt your Meniere's was getting worse?*

A: *Yes. Before I put self-help measures in place, I was in the grips of uncontrolled, unpredictable vertigo attacks. Meniere's was taking over my life.*

Q: *What do you mean by 'wooziness'?*

A: *I came up with the name 'wooziness' for the ongoing sense of imbalance. It was a mild dizziness that made me feel like an attack was imminent.*

Q: *What is a 'drop attack? Did you experience this?*

A: *I never had a drop attack. I understand there is a chance of suffering a 'drop attack', which is said to feel like "being suddenly pushed to the floor from behind."*

Q: *Did you ever have a Meniere attack while sleeping?*

A: *Yes. I experienced a number of vertigo attacks that woke me up from sleep.*

Q: *Is Meniere's disease worse in the morning or evening?*

A: *For me, it was often worse in the late afternoon.*

Q: *What is the Meniere's 'window of opportunity'?*

A: *The time between episodes where symptoms are*

manageable. This time period is what I call the 'window' of opportunity. A chance to do as much as you can towards your recovery. The time to do positive things for health: paying attention to diet, exercise, and reducing stress. One may not feel fantastic, but if you are careful, you can be productive and do normal day-to-day activities. The key is to maximize every opportunity to improve health.

ON THE QUESTION OF TINNITUS

Q: What is tinnitus?

A: It's the sensation of sound. You can even think the noise is outside your head, like buzzing going on around you. I initially went hunting for the origin of the sound, only to find the noise was inside me. It isn't just hearing damage that results in tinnitus; stress, doing too much, eating or drinking the wrong foods, loud environmental noise, can create what is called tinnitus.

Q: What causes tinnitus in Meniere's?

A: Tinnitus is due to damaged nerve hairs in the inner ear from Meniere attacks. Signals and vibrations from the nerve hairs are sent to the brain along the auditory nerve. The sound interpreted by the brain is described as 'a ringing across the brain'; the sound of tinnitus.

Q: Is increasing tinnitus always a warning of a vertigo?

A: For me, yes. A noticeable increase in tinnitus was always a warning. I'd notice a rise and increase in tinnitus when I was under stress, doing too much, eating or drinking the wrong foods, was overtired, or argued. Use tinnitus as an early warning sign, and back off your activities.

Q: Is tinnitus worse during a vertigo attack?

A: For me tinnitus increased before a vertigo attack. During an attack vertigo dominated me. I had no memory of tinnitus. However, other people do say tinnitus is markedly worse during the attack.

Q: Does tinnitus vary in sound?

A: Yes. There is a cacophony of sounds: ringing, hissing, static, crickets, screeching, whooshing, roaring, pulsing, ocean waves, buzzing, dial tones, and even music. The sound of chirping crickets is one of mine along with the 747 jet engine whine. At one time, the crickets seemed to pack themselves into the 747. One can have any of these sounds and two or more combinations is not uncommon.

Q: Can tinnitus affect both ears?

A: Tinnitus is brain activity and not the ear itself, but

yet, the constant ringing (or another sound) may seem like it is coming from one ear or both.

Q: *Is tinnitus the same for everyone?*

A: *I experienced tinnitus 24/7 and it only fluctuated louder before an attack. Other sufferers I spoke with experienced episodic tinnitus that went from extremely loud, to not loud enough to bother them.*

Q: *Do hearing aids help cure tinnitus?*

A: *No. Hearing aids help you to hear sounds, but they won't cure tinnitus. New technology hearing aids can include 'blue-tooth' programs to give specific relief from tinnitus, (such as a white noise sound), which helps to mask an element of tinnitus. There are also tinnitus specialists who offer help for tinnitus.*

Q: *How did you cope with tinnitus?*

A: *I used the sound of tinnitus as a warning of an impending attack, so I paid attention to tinnitus volume. It was useful in that regard and helped me feel positive towards tinnitus and therefore not distressed.*

Q: *Did you try an alternative treatment for tinnitus?*

A: *I tried white noise sounds on a CD and acupuncture, none of which helped. I found meditation or music, helped me* *forget the tinnitus. Even a half-hour break from the noise was a relief.*

Q: What seems to make tinnitus worse?

A: Salt. Caffeine. Alcohol. Spicy foods. Stress. Getting overtired. Thinking about tinnitus makes it seem louder.

Q: Can the Epley maneuver help with tinnitus?

A: No. The Epley maneuver can help ease positional vertigo, but won't do anything for tinnitus.

Q: What did you do that helped your tinnitus?

A: I accepted it for what it was. I stopped focusing on how bad it was. I realized the noise was not a threat or a danger to my physical person. The more I let go and accepted tinnitus, rather like a noisy neighbor, the easier tinnitus was to live with.

ON THE QUESTION OF THE SENSES

Q: What is aural fullness?

A: A feeling of pressure, discomfort and fullness sensation in the ears. It feels like your ear is plugged with cotton wool; sounds you hear become unclear: distant, distorted, tinny, far away and fuzzy.

Q: What causes aural fullness in the ears?

A: Episodic fluctuating aural fullness is thought to be due to the build-up of pressure in the inner ear, most often associated with the onset of an attack.

Q: Can you go deaf from Meniere's disease?

A: Yes. If you have unilateral Meniere's, the affected ear will lose some degree of hearing. There are varying levels of deafness found in the affected ear of Meniere sufferers. If you have bilateral Meniere's you will likely have extreme difficulty with your hearing, but hearing professionals can help with this.

Q: Why does Meniere's disease cause deafness?

A: The hearing loss is due to a sensorineural type of nerve deafness. During an attack, the cochlear hair cells of the inner ear become bathed in sodium and potassium, due to the sudden rupturing of the Reissner membrane. This rupturing occurs every time you have an attack. These hair cells are responsible for transmitting sound impulses to the brain. As they become damaged, so does your hearing facility in the affected ear.

Q: Does Meniere's disease cause conductive hearing loss?

A: No, conductive hearing loss happens when there is a problem in the middle ear. Meniere's hearing loss is a sensorineural hearing loss.

Q: Can you get high-frequency hearing loss?

A: Typically, the hearing loss in Meniere's is in the lower frequencies, usually associated with levels required for listening to speech.

Q: What is Meniere's disease unilateral hearing loss?

A: Hearing loss in one ear, the affected ear.

Q: *What is a sensorineural hearing loss?*

A: *Hearing loss, which occurs in the inner ear to the cochlea (the sensory hearing organ) or damage to the neural pathways of hearing (nerves). Damage in both or one of these areas is known as a sensorineural hearing loss.*

Q: *Is hearing loss permanent with Meniere's disease?*

A: *The intensity and range of hearing deterioration caused by Meniere's disease are different for everyone. But once Meniere's is advanced, your level of hearing loss becomes permanent.*

Q: *How much permanent hearing damage can you get?*

A: *Most people sustain moderate to severe hearing loss in the affected ear within 10 to 15 years of diagnosis.*

Q: *Can Meniere's disease hearing loss be prevented?*

A: *Unfortunately there is no known way to prevent the natural progression of hearing loss. It is important to protect the hearing you have in the 'good' ear by protecting your ears e.g. using power tools, listening to music with headphones. If the hearing is lost in one ear, you want the other one to be working well. This is an important piece of advice to note.*

Q: *Is hearing loss the same for everyone?*

A: No. Hearing loss varies from person to person. I lost hearing rapidly and soon became 90 percent deaf in the affected ear; other sufferers I spoke to tell me they lost hearing slowly, some never become totally deaf in the ear.

Q: Can you have Meniere's disease without hearing loss?

A: It is part of the condition, to lose part of your hearing permanently. Most Meniere sufferers experience permanent hearing loss to some degree, but this can be countered with an amazing range of technical hearing devices.

Q: What is the difference between Meniere's and BPPV?

A: Within the inner ear is a structure called the labyrinth with semicircular canals, which hold fluids that help monitor the position and rotation of your head. Benign Paroxysmal Positional Vertigo (BPPV) is vertigo which occurs with movements of the head such as lying down, turning over in bed, turning the head. The difference with BPPV and Meniere's disease is that Meniere's vertigo is not related to head position.

Q: What are 'crystals' in the ear?

A: The balance system in the inner ear has otolith organs that contain tiny crystals. These crystals can become dislodged for no known reason and 'float' into the semicircular canals. When this happens, this can cause intense dizziness *and a spinning sensation that lasts less than five minutes in Paroxysmal Positional Vertigo.*

Q: *Does the Epley maneuver work for Meniere's disease?*

A: *Epley works to help relieve vertigo symptoms in BPPV. However, Meniere's disease is sensorineural, not crystal related.*

Q: *Can you have Meniere's disease and otosclerosis?*

A: *Yes you certainly can. I had Meniere's disease in one ear and was also diagnosed with otosclerosis in the other; a problem with the stiffening of the small bones (ossicles). Otosclerosis prevents sound from passing through to the inner ear. The stiffening closes the hearing canal, so eventually, you can't hear in that ear. I unfortunately have otosclerosis in the left ear, (the one unaffected by Meniere's), due to cold water exposure scuba diving and surfing in early days. The ENT specialist said it was 'Murphy's law', meaning I was just plain unlucky to have otosclerosis in my good ear.*

Q: *Why do normal sounds appear incredibly loud?*

A: *This is caused by a condition called hyperacusis: a hypersensitivity to normal sounds. The ear loses its dynamic range of hearing. Dynamic range is the ear's ability to cope with quick shifts in sound levels.*

Q: How did loud noises affect you?

A: Yes. There are two things the human body never adapts to. Sudden noises and vertigo. The body will adapt to most other sensory changes but never to those two. Noise is so stressful for Meniere sufferers; it's listed by psychologists as a psychological stress.

Q: What did you do to cope with environmental sounds?

A: As I experienced more hearing loss, I found that normal environmental sounds appeared unbearably loud. Noise gave me frights, even sounds like someone shutting a window. No one else heard these sounds quite like I did. I had to tell my family and friends when places were too loud for me. We'd move to a quieter corner or go outside. I also used a protective hearing device, a custom made sound diffuser like musicians wear during live concerts. Soft foam earplugs for hearing protection, purchased from a drug store or chemist, also work well for this.

Q: Describe the recruitment phenomenon in Meniere's disease?

A: Another reason why normal sounds may be unbearable is the recruitment factor associated with hearing loss; this is an abnormal increase in the perception of loudness, even though the noise may be slight. Have you noticed the recruitment factor in a café? You're quietly sipping a decaffeinated latte and suddenly the waitress drops a stainless spoon onto the tile floor. You get a super-shock! That's the recruitment factor.

Q: *Can you experience ear pain?*

A: *Yes, you can. Although ear pain is not a symptom of Meniere's disease, aural fullness is. In some people, this fullness causes acute ear pain at times.*

Q: *Can Meniere's disease cause an ear infection?*

A: *No. Meniere's disease doesn't cause ear infections. Neither is Meniere's disease an ear infection. There can be a tendency to feel your ears are blocked up. Don't be tempted to dig the 'fullness' out with cotton buds! Remember the rule is: never put anything in your ear smaller than your elbow, unless it's a hearing aid.*

Q: *Can you wear hearing aids when you have Meniere's?*

A: *I was fitted for hearing aids when I began to notice a hearing loss in the early stages of Meniere's. However, because my hearing was fluctuating at the time, the hearing aids did not help me at all, in fact, I found the volume and sound input distressing. I did get the technician to make a pair of noise blocker aids to help protect the hearing I had and these helped to limit noise recruitment.*

Q: *What are grommets?*

A: *Grommets are small tubes, either 'T' shaped or shaped like a grommet, made of silicone or Teflon, which are inserted under anesthetic into the eardrum. Once inserted, this lets air into the middle air space with can affect pressure in the fluid compartments.*

Q: *Did you try grommets for Meniere's?*

A: *No. There is a lot of medical opinion that indicates grommets are not effective. I didn't want to take any risk with the hearing I had, or undergo any unnecessary medical procedures.*

Q: *What is cochlea in relation to Meniere's?*

A: *The cochlea is the hearing sense organ of the inner ear, which is divided into three chambers: two filled with a fluid called perilymph and one chamber with a fluid called endolymph. When the reissner membrane (that separates the perilymph and endolymph fluids) ruptures and the fluids mix, Meniere sufferers have an acute vertigo attack.*

Q: *How have you dealt with hearing the loss in your life?*

A: *After my hearing loss stabilized, I sought help from an audiologist and purchased two hearing aids (thankful for a government subsidy due to hearing as a disability). Hearing devices are small but costly, some as pricey as a* laptop depending on the technology. The affected ear required considerable volume whereas the other ear affected by otosclerosis responded well to much lower volume. I also asked my wife to not talk from the inside of a cupboard or from another room, which she never quite got the hang of.

Q: *Were you worried Meniere's would go to the other ear?*

A: *Yes of course. There is nothing you can do, but wait and see. It wasn't until the usual time limit of five years had passed, when bilateral Meniere's is most likely to happen, that I stopped worrying about bilateral as a possibility.*

Q: *What is the saddest thing about losing your hearing?*

A: *Knowing that it would never be found.*

Q: *What part do eyes play in Meniere's disease?*

A: *Meniere's affects eye movement (nystagmus) but this can vary considerably.*

Q: *What is Meniere's disease nystagmus?*

A: *A Meniere attack is accompanied by nystagmus. This is uncontrolled eye movement whereby both eyes flick to the affected side and then back to the other side. This movement it due to the affected ear sending mixed signals to the brain.*

Q: Does Meniere's disease affect vision?

A: No, it doesn't affect or damage your vision, but I advocate regular eye checks and suitable prescription glasses (if necessary) because eyestrain can cause fatigue/stress, which can be a trigger for vertigo attacks.

ON THE QUESTION OF FAMILY

Q: *Why is Meniere's called an invisible disease?*

A: *Meniere's disease is one of those invisible diseases because you can look 'normal' and don't look ill, unless you are heading for a vertigo attack or you have just had one.*

Q: *How does Meniere's disease impact on close relationships?*

A: *Meniere's disease can dominate family life. Love in a time of Meniere's will test relationship bonds. Patience, understanding, and empathy on both sides help to reduce stress and tension. The 'well' partner can feel quite alone when the one they love is having acute attacks. As normal patterns of your 'old' life alter, both of you must deal with the affects of chronic illness.*

Q: *What important advice would you give to a caregiver?*

A: *It is very important for the partner to take personal time for themselves to balance their role as the caregiver. They can live in a state of anxiety, especially as they are responsible for helping and running the home. It can be a lonely time for the caregiver. Unfortunately, those most affected by the patient's illness do not always receive the support and help they need at this time. It can also be a thankless task. I was so involved in the condition, I hardly remember all the support my wife gave me. Yet she gave up her freelance clients so she could be there for me.*

Q: *What makes Meniere's vertigo frightening?*

A: *Every vertigo attack is frightening and during an acute attack, you have difficulty responding to others. You use all your energies coping with the physical onslaught of the vertigo symptoms and trying to control panic.*

Q: *Why is it important to let the family know how you are feeling?*

A: *Since the acute symptoms of Meniere's disease are ongoing and episodic, it is important to explain to your family what is happens to you during Meniere's attacks. This helps them to understand and know what to do or not to do. They can't mind read. It's up to you to let then know.*

ON THE QUESTION OF FRIENDS

Q: How important were friends when you were sick?

A: Actually not as important as my close family unit. The occasional contact with friends was enough to not become isolated from society in general.

Q: How can friends understand Meniere's disease?

A: They need you to tell them what you are going through and how things are for you. Good friends are ones who check in with you and stay in touch. True friends don't forget friends.

Q: How can friends help with Meniere's?

A: Friends can include you in activities and accept that Meniere's can make you somewhat unreliable because you might be fine on the days when you accept an invitation, but then cancel out at the last minute. They need to make allowances and stay flexible, be understanding and not take last minute cancellations personally. But they need to keep including you in social activities. If they do not, it is very easy for you to become isolated.

Q: *Did you tell your friends what was wrong with you?*

A: *Eventually I told my close friends, mainly because they knew something was up with me. Still, not everyone knew I was ill. I am a private person and didn't disclose Meniere's to everyone. With hearing loss, I experienced a noticeable change in my ability and desire to socialize, especially in large groups.*

Q: *In what social situations were you most challenged?*

A: *Definitely communicating with groups of people. As my hearing deteriorated, I misheard a lot and the hearing impediment made it difficult to have an easy conversation. I am a reasonably intelligent man who likes to have a chat, but mishearing words and misinterpreting what people were saying, was a real disadvantage. At times I would repeat 'wrong' words and totally miss the gist of a conversation. This led to people leaving me out of the conversation. One of the most isolating times of my life, I think.*

Q: *If you felt bad at a social event, what did you do?*

A: *I would just slip away quietly.*

Q: *How did late nights affect you?*

A: *Often a late night would precede a vertigo attack. Late nights were something I avoided. I did everything to not get overtired. It took me a few years to stay up late enough to see a New Year in at midnight.*

ON THE QUESTION OF WORK AND FINANCES

Q: Should I let people know I have Meniere's?

A: Knowing what you are going through, helps them to be more caring and to make allowances. You can be clear about what you can and can't do. As the disease develops, so your colleagues need to be updated about changes you need to make to your working day. If you explain that you have Meniere's and how it affects you, your employers and/or colleagues, will hopefully show their supportive side. I didn't do this and I think it created confusion. In retrospect, I would tell them.

Q: Can you work with Meniere's disease?

A: Being able to be employed with Meniere's and still perform at the level you used to, can be a problem. The fact is, you simply won't be able to take the stress or workload at the same level. You may have to negotiate your way to a lesser position with fewer demands. Hopefully, you can come to arrangements, as being socially included and financially independent in a time of Meniere's is important.

Q: *How does Meniere's affect working life?*

A: *Meniere's brings a new set of criteria to your health and your earning capacity. If you ignore the impact Meniere's is having on your life, your situation could escalate to the negative. From experience, the beginning stage is the time to make significant decisions, to address changes Meniere's will bring, especially if you are the primary financial contributor to the family. Your health deficit may impact on your household, finances, and job. You must take all your living factors into account. If you do this with the help of family and professionals, your life won't fall into chaos, because of Meniere's. The ideal position is to take your hands off the controls, but still be in control. You can solicit help from your partner, business colleagues, friends, and family.*

Q: *Could you multi-task?*

A: *I struggled to multi-task. It was a big issue for me. I had to take one thing at a time and concentrate on one thing only. If I made a list of single tasks, I would avoid doing one task following another. I no longer had effective time management or multiplicity. Meniere's reduced that ability in the early stages.*

Q: Did you work with Meniere's disease?

A: Initially. When I was first diagnosed I tried to carry on as usual. At first, I tried to work but I had such a high power job, I quickly fell behind. As an owner of a business, I would sit through meetings with clients plus meet deadlines and then socialize with business in the evenings. I couldn't keep the pace up. I suffered so many debilitating Meniere's attacks, I soon ran out of excuses for absences.

Q: Were you able to continue to work due to Meniere's disease?

A: I wasn't able to go along in the tracks of my old life. After using up all my sick leave and vacation leave, I gave up work.

Q: Did you tell your work colleagues you had Meniere's?

A: No. I kept it to myself. Even when I left my position in the business, they were unaware of why I had to resign.

Q: Why did you feel you couldn't tell your business partners?

A: I didn't want to be seen as the weak link or socially handicapped or incapable. My ego, I suppose.

Q: Should you let colleagues know you have Meniere's?

A: I really think it is a good idea to let employers and people you work with know how this condition is affecting you. Looking back, I certainly wish I had done that.

Q: If you feel ill, how can you make important decisions?

A: You can't when you are in the attack cycle. Wait until you have a window of relative health and find help from professionals and people you trust. Look at one issue at a time and take the decision-making process slowly. Trust that you will always come up with suitable solutions.

Q: How can you maintain an income stream?

A: If you are self-employed, look at options, like cutting down hours even if it means taking less money and/or hire someone to help you. Face this issue head-on, define and clarify your position. If you are employed, use the support of professional people to advise you of your legal position and options within your employment. Cut back on superfluous expenses. Less outgoings can create a surprising financial buffer.

Q: Should you figure out your situation on your own?

A: My suggestion is to look around and seek advice on what to do from a variety of professional sources, arbitrators, counselors and medical specialists. Use more than one source. Then go and talk with your employer or partners.

Q: *Is income protection insurance helpful for Meniere's?*

A: *Socrates, the ancient Greek philosopher once said, "Security is the absence of awareness of danger." My philosophy is this. Every action has a reaction. Paddle your own canoe and don't rely on disability if you can help it. Make adjustments and keep control of your finances. Make sure you legally protect your existing assets. When you are a weak link, the law of the social jungle can be very aggressive and possibly take advantage.*

Q: *What is your advice to minimize the financial impact?*

A: *If I had fully understood Meniere's in the beginning, I would have taken time off work to restructure things, without it impacting and draining financial resources. A little less money, more time and careful planning will give you a chance to survive financially.*

Q: *What impact did Meniere's have on your career?*

A: *At the time, I was running a multi-million dollar company. Meniere's signaled the end. The symptoms were so severe. Had I not had Meniere's, I would still be working at an international level.*

Q: How did Meniere's change your life path?

A: I lost a successful business career because of Meniere's. Meniere's had a massive impact on the subsequent direction of my life. I countered this change by writing, painting, and appreciating what is most important to me these days: my health and family above all else. This is not groundbreaking news, but it seems to be the same for anyone who has suffered from severe illness.

ON THE QUESTION OF DISABILITY

𝒬: Is Meniere's disease a disability?

𝒜: I think it is. Meniere's disease physical issues and psychological effects including depression and/or anxiety.

𝒬: Does Meniere's disease qualify for disability benefits?

𝒜: At the time of writing, if you are disabled because of Meniere's disease and the condition is so severe it keeps you from working, you may be entitled to Social Security Disability benefits. In the US, Meniere's is on the list of medical conditions for immediate approval, providing all the testing they require has been done. In the UK, you may be able to apply for a grant for practical support to help you do your job. For those people affected by severe and frequent attacks, full time or even part-time work may not be possible, so you may be looking to the government for benefits and allowances. Depending on your symptoms, you may be entitled to Disability Living Allowance.

Q: Is there help with railway fares?

A: Yes, in the UK if you have a hearing impairment or wear a hearing aid, or, if you are on a disability benefit for Meniere's, you can apply for a Disabled Person's Railcard to receive a third off rail travel, underground rail and some designated ferries.

Q: What are the rules about driving with Meniere's?

A: With any balance disorder, you are required to let the Department of Vehicle Licensing know. There are rules about Vertigo Vs. Driving. The DVLA may temporarily revoke a driving license due to certain medical conditions. The law on driving may be different in other countries, but to make sure you are insured to drive with Meniere's. It pays to check the law and the fine print.

Q: What is a Meniere's disease blue badge?

A: In the UK, Blue Badges are an entitlement to disabled parking. Blue Badges are not limited only to drivers. They're given to an individual who may be the passenger or the designated driver.

Q: Did you wear a Meniere's disease medical bracelet?

A: No I didn't. An identity bracelet for me would be a constant reminder of illness. I couldn't see the real need for it because you don't go unconscious during an attack! For some people, this might make them feel more secure. Personally, I didn't support Meniere's merchandising such as key rings, coffee mugs or sweatshirt. I could think of nothing worse than walking around with a t-shirt saying I have Meniere's disease.

Q: How can people get Meniere's disease support?

A: Support comes from Meniere societies, Meniere forums, Meniere support groups, Meniere blog posts and reading as many books as you can find on the subject!

ON THE QUESTION OF MANAGING MENIERE'S

Q: *How did you manage Meniere's disease symptoms?*

A: *I took a self-help approach and looked at many factors including stress, diet, exercise, supplements and maintaining a positive attitude.*

Q: *What are triggers?*

A: *A trigger is something that causes certain symptoms to occur. I worked on a list of potential things that might affect my symptoms. I learned to recognize triggers that either induced attacks or made the attacks more intense. I worked on eliminating triggers. When I identified a trigger, I could avoid the trigger and over time this helped to reduce the number of attacks I was having. The attacks themselves became less intense and didn't last as long. Eventually, I* eliminated episodes of Meniere's disease and I attribute this partly to recognizing and working with triggers.

Q: *Explain the purpose of your Meniere's disease diary?*

A: *Pen and paper are mighty tools for recovery. In early days of diagnosis, I went out and bought a diary, tan leather. Just the simple act of journaling and writing in the diary daily, (without missing a day) gave me a great sense of being in control. Keeping a diary was the beginning of the self-monitoring and self-management needed to overcome Meniere's and get better.*

Q: *What did you write in your diary?*

A: *I wrote down what I did every day; this allowed me to go back after an attack and look at what I had done over the previous days. What had I been doing? What did I eat? What gave me stress? Did I drink alcohol? Argue? Have a late-night? I wrote down everything I could think of. I tried to figure out what might be causing the attacks. The list of possible triggers was long. I also wrote down: how long did the attack last; I looked at the time frames between attacks.*

Q: *Was your diary collection useful in your recovery?*

A: *Certainly. These diaries helped in my recovery. Even the simple act of self-reflection, self-observation and recalling what you do, helps to put you in charge of your life again.*

Q: After you were better, what happened to your diaries?

A: The material was extremely useful. It was a record of my life with Meniere's and proved to be useful in writing books on Meniere's. I could see clearly what I did to get better without surgery or invasive procedures. It was fundamentally apparent: there is a lot you can do to help yourself get better. I am a great believer that you can achieve anything you set your mind and heart on. My specialist encouraged me to write a book about self-management from a sufferers' point of view. Eventually, I took the manuscript into his office and he endorsed my first book. These days he is retired from his practice. I am grateful to him because he was upfront and honest and never pushed surgery, as being the cure. Now that I have written everything I found out, the notes are now gone and have been replaced by a series of books.

ON THE QUESTION OF A MENIERE'S DIET

Q: What food allergies did you have when diagnosed?

A: I have never suffered from any food allergies.

Q: What diet do you recommend for Meniere's disease?

A: I did follow the principles of the Zone Diet. I ate six small meals a day to keep blood sugar levels up; increased servings of vegetables, both raw and cooked and added flaxseed oil to my diet. I added more fresh fruit than The Zone Diet allowed though, so I didn't adhere to it strictly. I used The Zone Diet as a template for healthy eating: more fiber; less processed food; avoid empty carbohydrates; eat less fat; lean meat; less sugar and an abundance of fresh vegetables. Basically, it's that kind of healthy eating style... without salt.

Q: *Did you follow The Paleo Diet?*

A: *Paleo was not in vogue when I was diagnosed, but I inadvertently followed their recommendations for grains, low sugar, and salt, (no salt and no simple sugars) less processed foods and healthy whole foods.*

Q: *What are general rules for food and Meniere's?*

A: *Eat well-balanced meals. Don't skip meals. Eat energy-boosting snacks (low fat, low sugar, low salt snacks). Severely limit salt, alcohol, and caffeine. Eat fresh fruit and vegetable and less processed foods.*

Q: *Why is a low salt diet recommended for Meniere's disease?*

A: *Sodium creates fluid retention and as such creates an imbalance in the body's fluids, especially in the inner ear. This can trigger vertigo. So one goal for managing Meniere's vertigo is to reduce the total body fluid volume by avoiding substances that may trigger or exacerbate fluid pressure build up in the inner.*

Q: *What is a low sodium diet for Meniere disease?*

A: *According to the University of Maryland Medical Centre, maintaining a low salt diet involves restricting sodium intake to between 1,500 to 2,000 milligrams per day. I would aim for between 500 to 1000 mg per day.*

Q: *What low salt measures did you take?*

A: *Adding salt may be the first habit you give up. There is plenty of sodium occurring naturally in foods. Maintain a low salt intake on a daily basis. Avoid adding salt to food while cooking. Don't add salt to meals at the table. Throw away the saltshaker. One of the best ways to change a habit is to not buy any salt or salted foods or bring them into the house. When eating out, I asked for no salt and avoided meals with sauces. I learned to read food information on the backs of packets and bottles. Initially I kept a tally of my salt intake every day until I educated myself on ingredients and their salt content.*

Q: *Can you cut out all salt?*

A: *Possibly, but zero sodium is not necessary or advisable. Don't try to eliminate salt altogether; your muscles and nerves need it to function. For more information, talk to a dietician or nutritionist.*

Q: *Where are 'hidden' salts found in foods?*

A: *A general low salt rule, avoid or limit processed foods that are high in sodium, canned vegetables, soups, spaghetti sauce, most sauces in fact...ketchup, vegetable juices, and ready-to-eat cereals. Avoid high salt foods like canned ravioli, salted nuts, potato crisps, broth, bouillon cubes, and gravies. The list goes on. Initially look at what you normally eat. You* will be surprised when you run a salt count over your food intake.

Q: *How can I shop low salt?*

A: *Many choices of low salt foods are available in supermarkets, food stores, and markets. It's easy to replace high salt foods with low salt foods. Here's an example. Instead of crackers with a high salt content, choose a brand with the lowest salt content and look at how much salt is contained in every 100gm. You can still eat foods you love, you just have to change the brands and put low salt packets, cans or cartons into your shopping trolley.*

Q: *Can you still eat out and do take-outs?*

A: *Yes you can, but you need to ask for no salt or MSG when you order and avoid dishes with sauces, like black bean sauce, soy sauce and chili sauce in Asian restaurants. Don't reach for the sauces.*

Q: *What is the difference between sodium and salt?*

A: *Sodium is a chemical name for salt. Wherever you see sodium listed in ingredients, sodium means salt: sodium bicarbonate, sodium nitrate (which is a preservative). There are many different types of salt: iodized, sea salt, Himalaya pink salt, plain salt. The amount of salt in food is listed as sodium on the label.*

Q: *How much salt in a low salt diet?*

A: *You know you need to eat healthily on a low salt diet but how do you do it? Well, the first thing is to know how much daily sodium (salt) intake there is on a low salt diet. A low salt diet is 400 - 1000 mgs of salt a day. A normal salt diet is 1100 – 3300 mgs a day. A high salt diet is 4000 - 6000 mgs a day. Maintaining a sodium intake below 2000 mgs a day takes effort. Initially, you can try to reduce salt levels to 1000 - 2000 mgs a day and see if there is any improvement. You may be fine at that level or you can reduce it to 500 -1100 mgs a day. There is no need to be afraid of salt; you just need to control the intake. To maintain a low salt diet, you need to read the Nutritional Information printed by law, on the side of cans and packets of food.*

Q: *Is there an easy way to adopt a low salt diet?*

A: *Throw away the saltshaker! Adapting to a low salt diet is a key element in reducing symptoms.*

Q: *Did you juice for Meniere's disease?*

A: *Yes. Lemon, orange and lime juice for my vitamin C. Beetroot, celery, apples, and carrots create delicious vitamin-rich juices.*

Q: *What about sugar and Meniere's?*

A: *Simple sugars are 'bad' sugars. Because almost as*

soon as you eat them, they cause a sudden spike, (sugar high) followed by a sudden drop in blood sugar levels. This sudden spike and drop are thought to be a possible trigger for a Meniere's vertigo attack. To lower the level of blood sugar in your body, it is important to cut out simple carbohydrates and simple sugars from your diet. Instead, go for complex carbohydrates, which are known to stabilize the body's blood sugar levels.

Q: What foods should you avoid with Meniere's disease?

A: The following foods should be reduced or eliminated from your diet: concentrated fruit juice, candy, cookies, biscuits, cakes, muffins, donuts, sweets, pasta and bread made with white flour, sugary cereals, white sugar, ice cream, milk chocolate (go for dark chocolate). No jams. No soda drinks. Pre-made sauces. Everything preserved with salt, such as olives and tinned fish. Most cheeses. Our modern diet and processed foods all have added salt.

Q: What foods should you eat with Meniere's disease?

A: Basically whole primary foods. Whole grain bread, brown rice, legumes like dried beans, pulses and lentils, vegetables, barley, wild rice, soybeans, fruits, nuts and seeds, fish and meat. All of these complex carbohydrates have multiple benefits and give you more energy. Not only do they taste great, they're a great way to get the minerals and vitamins your body needs to heal.

Q: *What was your favorite low salt meal?*

A: *Thin Italian spaghetti with a simmered sauce of Roma tomatoes, olive oil, garlic and topped with ground black pepper and topped with shredded fresh basil picked straight from the herb garden.*

Q: *What oils did you use?*

A: *I cooked with virgin coconut oil and olive oil. I used cold-pressed extra virgin olive oil and flaxseed oil in dressings. I also ate oily fish giving me a high intake of Omega-3.*

Q: *Did you enjoy cooking for Meniere's?*

A: *Yes. I have a great love of good food. I cooked a lot of Italian style dishes I adapted for low salt. Cooking was great occupational therapy with very tasty outcomes.*

Q: *What kitchen equipment did you use?*

A: *A barbecue, indoor grill and hotplate griddle, terracotta pizza stone for the oven, blender, juicer and most important: good quality, sharp-bladed kitchen knives.*

Q: *Did Meniere's affect your weight?*

A: *No, not at all. I maintained a healthy weight through exercise, despite the early stages of couch potato! I would always get up when I could and go for walks.*

Q: *Are bananas good for Meniere's disease?*

A: *Bananas are one of the richest sources of potassium and a convenient food source. Potassium-rich foods help the body control salt levels.*

Q: *How does potassium help Meniere's disease?*

A: *Potassium helps relieve blood pressure, anxiety and stress, improve water balance, and assist the nervous system. These are all essential functions affected by Meniere's. Many people take diuretics and unless the medication is specifically 'potassium-sparing', taking of diuretics daily can cause potassium depletion in the body. Adding bananas to your diet can help.*

Q: *What about gluten and Meniere's?*

A: *During my recovery, I followed a healthy diet of whole foods but did not reduce or eliminate gluten.*

Q: *What about plant sterols?*

A: *Eating well to get well involves using anti-inflammatory foods in your diet. Young green shoots of alfalfa, mung beans, and cress are all rich in plant sterols. By adding sprouts to your diet, you reduce inflammation. You can improve the circulation to the head and inner ear by using regenerative nutrition, such as plant sterols, which help alleviate the symptoms of Meniere's disease.*

Q: *Is ginger good for Meniere's disease?*

A: *Ginger boosts the immune system. I found ginger tea, made with grated ginger root and boiling water helped to control the woozy feeling. Adding ginger to your diet helps to raise and balance the energy assisting circulation. Ginger was prized by spice traders for centuries and is believed to promote vitality and a long life. Ginger acts as an antiemetic, to help with nausea. Check with your doctor first if you are taking blood thinner medication.*

Q: *Are there natural diuretics for Meniere's disease?*

A: *There are many foods that have a diuretic effect, such as apple cider vinegar, artichoke, asparagus, beets, Brussel sprouts, cabbage, carrots, cranberry juice, cucumber, green tea, fennel, lettuce, oats and watermelon.*

Q: *Can green tea help with Meniere's disease?*

A: *Green tea is a natural diuretic and contains powerful antioxidants and bioflavonoids which are valuable to the Meniere's diet.*

Q: *What was your worst dining out experience?*

A: *Chinese chicken wonton soup. I asked for no salt with my order. The steaming noodle bowl arrived with wontons, but the broth tasted like oily bathwater. Without the usual MSG or salt, the dish tasted ghastly.*

ON THE QUESTION OF CAFFEINE

Q: Does caffeine affect Meniere's?

A: Caffeine has been shown to raise the body's blood volume and cause small blood vessels to constrict. This reduces the blood supply to the inner ear while causing a build-up of inner ear pressure and fullness. Because of its effect on the cerebral vascular system, caffeinated coffee can increase tinnitus levels and is a known trigger for causing Meniere attacks.

Q: Did you have to give up coffee?

A: Initially, that is exactly what I had to do. I gave up drinking caffeinated coffee and switched to decaffeinated coffee, (5 mg of caffeine a serving).

Q: What was your favorite beverage?

A: Hot drinks like fresh lemon juice or lime, with a teaspoon of honey, in hot water. Also herbal teas. There are delicious tisanes available that use teas combined with spices and fruit, such as green tea and ginger.

Q: Is there caffeine in medications?

A: Yes. Caffeine can be produced synthetically and added to medications. If you are cutting down your caffeine intake, be aware that some non-prescription drugs such as a headache and pain reliever tablets can contain 65 mg of caffeine in a tablet. Product labels are required to list caffeine in the ingredients but not required to state the actual amount of the substance.

Q: Is there caffeine in certain foods and drink?

A: Yes. It's not just coffee that contains caffeine. Green tea has 25-40 mg of caffeine in a cup; black tea 40-70 mg; cocoa 5 mg per teaspoon; a sweet chocolate bar 1.45 oz. contains 27 mg. Red Bull 8.5 oz. contains 80 mg; Coca-Cola Classic 12oz has 34.5 mg of caffeine, Diet Coke 46.5 mg; Pepsi-Cola, 37.5 mg.

Q: Do you drink coffee, now you are better?

A: Yes. I'd bought an Italian coffee machine made of solid brass with an eagle perched on top. The eagle sat there and lost its shine while waiting for the day when I would *flick the red switch and fire him up. That day came. Now I'm back enjoying lattes, flat whites, and espressos. Yes! Finally the Italian, Brazilian, Columbian and Arabica are back in my blood. I do limit them to a maximum of two cups of coffee a day.*

ON THE QUESTION OF ALCOHOL

Q: *Does alcohol affect Meniere disease?*

A: *Alcohol can cause the blood vessels to contract, which restricts the blood supply to your inner ear. Surprisingly though, small amounts of alcohol, such as a glass of red wine or half a pint of beer a day, can help peripheral circulation. In the early stages, I didn't drink any alcohol. Now my alcohol consumption is 2 or 3 glasses a week.*

Q: *Why should you cut down or avoid alcohol?*

A: *Alcohol affects both your balance and your vascular system. The more your drink, the less stable you feel and your blood pressure will rise. Using alcohol as a way to alleviate stress is not helpful.*

Q: *Do you drink alcohol now you are better?*

A: *Yes, but always in moderation. For health, I don't go over the recommended daily units and I never binge drink.*

ON THE QUESTION OF SUPPLEMENTS

Q: Why are nutritional supplements used for Meniere's?

A: Tests revealed that Meniere sufferers are usually low in iron, low in vitamin A and either high or low in sodium, low or high in potassium and low or high in magnesium and low in Co-enzyme Q_{10}.

Q: What would you recommend as supplements?

A: To assist healing, it is essential to supply all the nutrients and minerals the body requires. The first supplement to invest in, is always a quality daily multi-vitamin.

Q: Did you read up on vitamins and minerals?

A: Yes. As well as talking to nutritional therapists, I read books like 'Optimum Sports Nutrition' by Michael Colgan.

One of many informative books on nutrition I read. The more you understand how important minerals and vitamins are for your general wellbeing, the more you'll be able to help yourself to maximum health.

Q: *Do you think supplements helped in your recovery?*

A: *I really believe so. In the early stages of Meniere's, my body was deficient in vitamins and my adrenals were down. I thought if I was going to step up my physical goals and improve my health, I needed to look at my vitamin and mineral intake, which I did. This was a general health interest though, not an obsession!*

Q: *Is the quality and source of supplements important?*

A: *Certainly, I always read the small print to check the actual quantity of minerals and vitamins.*

Q: *Supplements are expensive, how did you counter this?*

A: *I bought in bulk with good discounts from a reputable supplement importer who delivered to my house. She was a nutrition expert who had recovered from a chronic condition using vitamins and supplements for healing, so she shared a lot of information.*

Q: *What was your personal supplement regime?*

A: *With the help and guidance of nutritional*

professionals and product information from health and wellness companies, I worked out the following personal vitamin and supplement regime to get better. Note that this was my personal regime and as with any vitamin and mineral supplementation it is advisable to talk with your doctor first. I have included the amounts and the reason for taking these specific ones to support the body during Meniere's. Many sufferers ask me for Meniere Man's supplement regime, so I have included it here for you.

1. *Vitamin C*: *Vitamin C 2000 mg to 4000 mg spread throughout the day and at least one hour before or after food. Vitamin C increases blood vessel permeability and allows red cells to mobilize. Vitamin C supports the kidneys, liver and immune system.*

2. *Vitamin E*: *Increases blood vessel health and permeability, promotes healing and is an antioxidant. 400 mg of vitamin E, twice a day, at meal times.*

3. *EFA's*: *Essential fatty acids are important for reducing inflammation and assisting in nerve transmission. Take a 300 mg salmon oil capsule, three times a day. Or flaxseed oil one teaspoon, three times a day.*

4. *Complex Vitamin B*: *Clinically proven to assist the nervous system helping reduce stress, depression, relieve tension, generally picking up your energy levels and keeping your immune system supported. Complex B's assist nerve* regeneration. B12 works to alleviate dizziness caused by a deficiency of this essential vitamin. B Complex supplements contain B6, B2, B5, B12, plus a balance of essential minerals. Take one complex B supplement, at lunch with food.

5. Multivitamin: once a day. When you take a multivitamin, you need to read the levels of vitamins in it and take that into account when you add the supplements you are taking. Choose a scientifically formulated multi-vitamin of high quality. Twin Labs, Swisse Men, Swisse Women. All are documented to be high-quality sources of vitamins and minerals. When you take a quality supplement, you can feel the difference.

6. Potassium Sulfate: replenishes potassium depletion in the body and helps maintain your body's fluid levels. It works with sodium in all cells including nerve synapses to maintain or restore membrane potential and assist metabolic processes; 85 mg once a day.

7. Calcium supplement: containing Pantothenate 75 mg, Calcium Citrate 200 mg for bone support. May support cochlear bone by preventing bone depletion and osteoporosis. Calcium assists with sleep. A glass of warm milk with a teaspoon of honey before bed helps you sleep.

8. Magnesium Citrate: 50 mg. Supports the nervous system.

Q: *You had two vitamin and supplement regimes. Can you explain?*

A: *Illness, medication, stress, anxiety increase your body's need for essential minerals and vitamins. This means you need to give your system a boost with additional supplements for three-month periods, throughout the year. I also took additional vitamins that provided extra support for my adrenal glands and immune system all year.*

Q: *What was your three-month booster regime?*

A: *In the early stages of Meniere's, in addition to the daily vitamin regime, I would use the following supplements for a three month period. Then I would go back to my basic daily vitamin regime.*

1. Zinc: *daily. Strengthens the immune system. Improves cognitive function and promotes increased energy.*

2. Oil of Primrose: *daily. EFA (essential fatty acid) Boosts your immune system and supports your nervous system.*

3. Selenium: *-daily. Keeps blood vessels healthy, reduces anxiety and depression; improves the immune system.*

4. Carnitine: *daily. A natural antioxidant; helps mood, memory, and cognitive ability; helps control blood sugar levels.*

5. *Chromium:* *daily. 30 mg helps control cholesterol.*

6. *Co-enzyme Q10:* *- 50 mg, three times a day for 90 days; helps improve vertigo symptoms and strengthens the immune system; helps prevent dizziness; provides energy; assists memory, mood and builds resistance to stress, infection, and disease.*

7. *Silica:* *Encourages self-repair and healing to the immune and nervous systems. Facilitates the electrical balance of the cells; helps regenerate the liver and repair the body. Liquid silica three times a day for three months.*

Q: *Do you still take vitamins and mineral supplements?*

A: *I now just concentrate on eating a healthy diet with plenty of essential oils. But if my body is under stress, I take my booster regime.*

Q: *Did you try ginkgo biloba?*

A: *Ginkgo is known to have a beneficial action on circulation, especially to the arterial circulation of the head. Ginkgo supplement is said to decrease tinnitus and dizziness by increasing blood flow to the head and therefore increasing circulation of the middle ear. I was recommended to try two capsules, three times a day for two months to see if it helped my symptoms. I didn't recognize any change in my body when*

I took it. If you take ginkgo, do not take with aspirin. Be sure to check with your doctor first.

Q: Is medical cannabis used to treat Meniere's disease symptoms?

A: Medical cannabis can help well over 100 illnesses and diseases. However, my ENT specialist told me early on in my diagnosis, never to be involved in anything that affects your balance and so I haven't. I avoided (and still do) substances that remotely affect stability or balance, raise blood pressure, or may contain contaminants or unknown additives.

Q: Do you think vitamin D helps?

A: Vitamin D is essential for health. The best source of vitamin D is a 15-minute dose of sunshine. Sunlight in the morning is the best when it is called blue light. When you go for a walk, sunlight is absorbed through your eyes and becomes Vitamin D in your body, so it's important not to wear sunglasses, or sunblock for 15 minutes in morning.

Q: What supplements, if any, can help with tinnitus?

A: Magnesium supplements may help relieve tinnitus associated with Meniere's disease.

ON THE QUESTION OF ALTERNATIVE THERAPIES

Q: Which alternative medicine treatments did you try?

A: I used a combination of natural therapies to help symptoms. Mind-body medicine such as breathing techniques, biofeedback, and meditation with and without guided imagery, total body relaxation techniques, massage, therapy, acupressure, and acupuncture. Each and every alternative therapy comes down to a personal choice. There is no 'one size fits all' with therapies. What gives relief and comfort to one person, may do the opposite for another. I don't advocate any one therapy. I do say do your research first and only use a registered practitioner.

Q: What helped you most?

A: While I tried different therapies, once or twice, these are the therapies I decided to do on a regular basis.

1. *Biofeedback:* *to learn about tension and stress I was holding in my body. I had two sessions initially.*

2. *Meditation:* *ocean waves, guided verbal meditations, meditation music. I bought four CDs and rented others from the library every fortnight.*

3. *Breathing:* *for total body relaxation. I learned and then practiced this at home.*

4. *Acupuncture:* *with a Doctor of Chinese Medicine. I went once a week for four sessions, then every two weeks for the following month. After that, when I felt like it.*

5. *Massage:* *acupressure with a therapist, once a week for a while, then every two weeks, then once a month.*

Q: *What is the upper cervical chiropractic for Meniere's disease?*

A: *A treatment to correct vertebra in the spine that are misaligned through a traumatic injury, such as a motor vehicle crash. The theory is once these misalignments are treated, (a gentle tap to unlock the vertebrae with no cracking, popping or twisting during the correction) the body can function optimally and self-heal. I am not advocating this practice because I avoid neck manipulations.*

Q: *What one piece of advice would you give?*

A: Many natural therapists I spoke with stressed one point: avoid any neck manipulations, so I stuck to that. Even when having sports massages I asked therapists to leave the neck area alone. Also be selective, use your powers of deduction and analysis. Research the pros and cons of the practices you may be considering.

Q: Did you have massage therapy?

A: Yes, but not just before or just after an attack! During remission times, massage can help increase circulation, reduce fluid buildup, relaxation and stress relief. This may collectively help reduce the number of attacks.

Q: What is cranial-sacral therapy?

A: The therapy has its origins in osteopathy, and it involves the rebalancing of the craniosacral system through gentle, non-invasive manipulation of the cranium, and the bones of the face and spine.

Q: What is osteopathy therapy?

A: Osteopathy treatment (OT) may be a positive complementary medicine for the four defining symptoms of Meniere's; by improving the function of abnormal tissues in the head, cervical, thoracic and TMJ areas and provide symptomatic relief. Chiropractors or osteopaths may adjust the head, jaw, and neck to relieve movement restrictions that could affect the inner ear. People have asked me about this therapy, but it was not part of my management plan.

Q: What is kinesiology?

A: Applied kinesiology (AK) uses muscle strength testing to identify nutritional deficiencies and health problems. Weakness in certain muscles corresponds to specific diseases or body imbalances. Research suggests that Meniere's vertigo may improve with rotational exercises. However, this is still in the early stages of research, it is not a common alternative therapy as yet.

Q: What is cranial osteopathy?

A: Craniosacral therapists use their hands to gently move bones of the skull to relieve pressure on the head. This is thought to help the nervous system function better and allow fluids to move better inside the head.

Q: Can acupuncture help Meniere's disease symptoms?

A: The World Health Organization (WHO) lists Meniere's disease as one of 104 conditions that can be treated effectively with acupuncture. There are specific acupuncture ear points, kidney, sympathetic, occiput, heart, and adrenal, which may help relieve dizziness associated with Meniere's disease. Chronic cases of Meniere's may be treated at the body points on the spleen, triple warmer and kidney meridians.

Q: Did you try acupuncture?

A: Yes. It really did help. After every session with acupuncture with a registered practitioner, I felt better.

Q: Can acupressure massage help with symptoms?

A: Acupressure massage works on restoring the flow of energy by applying pressure to specific acupressure points during a massage. I felt it did help my symptoms of extreme tiredness. There are other symptoms that acupuncture focuses on, for example, P6 or Pericardium 6, a point located three finger-breaths below the wrist, is an effective acupressure point that relieves vertigo and associated symptoms like nausea. GV 20 or Governing Vessel 20 is a powerful acupressure point for vertigo, located at the center of the top of the head. Acupressure point GB 21 or Gall Bladder 21 relieves dizziness, vertigo, nausea and motion sickness; this point is located on both shoulders.

Q: Can Reiki help with Meniere's disease symptoms?

A: Reiki uses a technique commonly referred to as palm healing or hands-on healing. According to practitioners, the healing effects are mediated by channeling the universal energy known as qi (pronounced "chi"). This energy permeates our bodies but is not measurable by modern scientific techniques. It is thought to help relaxation, assist in the body's natural healing processes and develop emotional, mental and spiritual well-being. I liked this therapy.

Q: *Can reflexology help Meniere's disease symptoms?*

A: *Reflexology is reported to help in treating the symptoms of vertigo by restoring your body to a balanced energy flow. It works on a specific set of pressure points, located in various parts of the body: cervical spine, ear, neck, hands, and feet.*

Q: *Are there any alternative treatments or remedies?*

A: *Ginkgo may help relieve tinnitus in some people. Fenugreek tea (steeped in cold water) is known to stop cricket noises and ringing in the ears. Chamomile tea promotes relaxation and helps with sleep. Relaxation techniques can be beneficial: biofeedback, yoga, massage and meditation of all kinds.*

Q: *Can wearing Sea Bands on the wrist help nausea?*

A: *Yes, they can help sometimes. Sea Bands are two small stretchy bands made of a thick knitted fabric and a small plastic marble, reusable and you can purchase these from drug stores. Place one on each wrist, the ball applies pressure to the acupressure points on the wrists.*

Q: *Did you take any homeopathic treatments?*

A: *Yes. I used homeopathy a lot as part of my self-help* *program. Homeopathy helps with anxiety and depression. I used Arnica drops taken in a small glass of water, to take the shock out of my body after an Meniere's vertigo attack.*

Q: *Did you use Bach Flower remedies?*

A: *I used a remedy called Rescue Remedy after a vertigo attack. I found that helped give me some bounce back and took some of the stress away after vertigo attacks.*

Q: *What specific aromatherapy oils did you use?*

A: *I used a variety such as Clary Sage, Tangerine, Sweet Orange, Sweet Basil or Holy Basil, Frankincense or Sacred Frankincense; mainly a few drops in the bath as oils. Some I burned in oil burners for the general atmosphere.*

Q: *Does the quality of aromatherapy oil make a difference?*

A: *They must be pure essential oils with no additives from a reputable company. I used oils from The Tisserand Institute in The United Kingdom. They offer educational material of essential oils, and their safe usage, based on genuine evidence, scientific data, and credible research.*

Q: *How did you use essential oils?*

A: *I added six drops of selected oil into a warm bath — used oils in a diffuser, or an essential oil burner in the living* room, and bedroom. Oils are for external use only and, if used for massage, must be diluted in a carrier oil, such as almond oil; never use directly on the skin.

Q: *What aromatherapy oils helped with vertigo?*

A: *While I can't say categorically that aromatherapy oils did or didn't help with vertigo, they did help me feel calmer and relaxed at home. They added a degree of comfort and a sense of well-being.*

Q: *What is ginger oil helpful for?*

A: *Ginger is used for nausea, but is also effective in relieving dizziness and vertigo by increasing circulation to the brain.*

Q: *What is lavender oil helpful for?*

A: *Lavender is commonly used for relief of stress, anxiety, and depression, and is effective for dizziness.*

Q: *Is peppermint good for vertigo relief?*

A: *Peppermint is highly effective for vertigo and nausea. Rose is effective for depression, vertigo, and relaxation.*

ON THE QUESTION OF HEALTH AND FITNESS

Q: Have you always been interested in sport?

A: Yes, I've always been actively involved in sports and fitness activities since a young boy, when I was a keen national surfer at competition level and on the swim team.

Q: Did this stop with Meniere's?

A: At the time I was diagnosed I was an advanced level scuba diver. I had to give this up as diving and Meniere's are just not compatible. I replaced diving with windsurfing. I also became more regular with my daily walking routine.

Q: Does Meniere's limit physical activity?

A: You can't do much when you have a vertigo attack. On the other hand, after an attack, you can do most anything.

There is a golden opportunity, a window that you should open after an attack. Literally, let the fresh air and light in. Do as much as you can without overdoing things and exhausting yourself. Remember, the more you do, the more you can do. Move forward to recovery.

Q: *Does exercise help Meniere disease?*

A: *Yes. On so many levels, from increasing general fitness and balance to helping with recovery and maintaining a positive mental state.*

Q: *How soon after a vertigo attack would you do exercise?*

A: *As soon as I could. Walking, tai chi and anaerobic core training are all excellent for balance training. You can take up racquetball, tennis, basketball, volleyball or any sport that interests you. Check with your doctor about how often and for how long you should exercise.*

Q: *Did you push your physical limits?*

A: *Always. You have to push forward. Every incremental step is an achievement, no matter how small. When you exercise more, you notice you can lift a little more, walk a little further and balance better. That is how it goes.*

Q: *How frequently did you exercise?*

A: *At the very least I walked every day if I wasn't*

having a vertigo attack or the first day recovering from one.
I tried to do gym five days a week. On the weekends I would
do a sport like windsurfing if I could.

Q: Did you exercise on bad days?

A: On 'bad days' I would do small steps, like walk
around the garden or take a stroll along the road. I found
bad days difficult because I always got a feeling of having a
setback and I had to work with myself to not give up and tell
myself, what mattered was the bigger recovery picture. I had
to get the focus right and not get down about attacks or bad
days. If you don't exercise, you will find most days are bad
days.

Q: Did exercise make you feel better?

A: Yes, as long as I didn't go overboard and get tired.

Q: When did you feel a sense of relief from symptoms?

A: I often felt relief from many of the symptoms when I
was on holiday, by the sea, in the countryside and when doing
sports activities. The meditation and aromatherapy baths
helped as well.

Q: Is boxing good for Meniere's?

A: Fitness boxing where you hit a punching bag, stretch,
and do strength training helps improve muscle strength,

balance, stamina, and eye-hand coordination. Boxing with another, I wouldn't recommend.

Q: *What is your pick of physical activities for Meniere's disease?*

A: *Walking and core training exercises. Both were essential to my recovery.*

Q: *Why is walking good?*

A: *Getting out of the house in the fresh air and walking freely, is essential to living a healthy, independent life. Staying inside can lead to a downward spiral. After vertigo attacks, as soon as you are able, get up and go for a walk, even if it's just to the lamp-post. Regular exercise is key to maintaining and increasing circulation, strength, flexibility, balance, and endurance, as well as keeping depression away. Taking steps to walk on a regular basis helps improve balance. Walking in the sunshine increases vitamin D and maintains bone strength and makes you less likely to take a fall.*

Q: *What was your best form of exercise?*

A: *Definitely walking. It was easy, simple and didn't require anything much in the way of equipment except good shoes. I challenged myself with distance and pace.*

Q: *What was your least preferred form of exercise?*

A: Tennis, because I'm no good at backhand anyway.

Q: Can you go running with Meniere's?

A: Keen runners often ask this question. I would suggest if running is your sport, go for it. If you feel unstable, walk or jog on those days and go running on the good days.

Q: What are the two physical activities you gave up?

A: Theme parks rides and scuba diving.

Q: What sports can't you do with Meniere's?

A: Flying or gliding a plane, scuba diving.

Q: Did you take up new physical activities?

A: Yes I did. Try was the word. I tried skiing and took up snowboarding, tried wakeboarding, but spent more time windsurfing, learned to weightlift light to medium weight and relearned surfing.

Q: What was the most daring thing you did?

A: Go up a ski gondola in high winds and ski downhill in a whiteout. Note, I didn't attempt this on a 'bad day'!

Q: What tested the limit of your sense of balance?

A: High places. Shopping malls, balconies, glass lifts, the *edge of cliffs, stairwells.*

Q: You took up a lot of balance activities? Why?

A: I needed to develop my balance sensors, which proved to be right for me.

Q: Why are balance exercises so important?

A: Balance exercises also gave me confidence. When you lose your balance, you lose confidence. I never imagined I would get back to normal; let alone learn to snowboard and windsurf while I was suffering the symptoms of Meniere's. Yet, it was these balancing activities that helped me regain my equilibrium and ultimately recovered a full life.

Q: Can balance exercises help Meniere's?

A: Tai chi, yoga, physical therapy, muscle strengthening, stretching, can all help with balance. This, in turn, gives you the confidence to try new things plus your general health improves with any exercise.

Q: Is core balance good for Meniere's?

A: The core muscles are in the hips, back, and abdomen. Strengthening these muscles helps with coordination of the central nervous system.

Q: Are stretching exercises good for Meniere's disease?

A: Definitely. A stretching program for muscles of the calves, hamstrings, hip flexors, quadriceps, shoulders, and lower back helps to improve your range of motion and balance. When you have Meniere's, your body is in a constant state of balancing and this creates tension especially in the neck and shoulders. I did stretching exercises three or four times per week.

Q: Are there vestibular balance exercises for Meniere's disease?

A: Yes there are. Vestibular rehabilitation (VR), or vestibular rehabilitation therapy (VRT) is an exercise program designed to help reduce vertigo and dizziness. A series of specific exercises based on three principal methods of exercise can be prescribed, where the brain learns to ignore the abnormal signals it is receiving from the inner ear.

Q: Can you do yoga with Meniere's disease?

A: Yes, you can do yoga on 'good days'. With any physical activity, you need to listen to your body. Attempt what you feel comfortable with.

Q: Why is yoga good?

A: Yoga postures and breathing help reduce tension in the muscles and improve flexibility, strengthening and stretching muscles, essential for balance. Yoga challenges static balance, the ability to stand in one spot without swaying, and dynamic balance, the ability to anticipate and react to changes as you move. Breathing and meditation reduce stress, and helps with relaxation.

Q: Why is tai chi good?

A: Tai chi uses a series of slow-flowing motions, and involves learning and memorizing new skills and movement patterns while practicing deep, slow breathing. This ancient Eastern exercise uses the conscious control to improve balance, flexibility and the mind.

Q: What was your favorite winter sports?

A: Snowboarding.

Q: What were your favorite summer sports?

A: Windsurfing with my daughter. Swimming at the beach. Relaxing in a hammock.

Q: What were your favorite family activities?

A: Family holidays. All the school events.

Q: Did you ever go away with friends?

A: Yes. My good friend Al came over from Whistler, Canada and I took him to remote rivers to go fishing for wild brown trout. I didn't tell him I was suffering from Meniere's and he never guessed. We drove on winding interior roads and I had a whole week free of symptoms. Times like that were great for my sense of wellbeing and confidence. Although I had Meniere's, I was still spending time doing what I wanted. I tried to make the most of the opportunities, rather than miss out on life.

Q: *What was your greatest physical challenge?*

A: *A week's snowboarding vacation with the family in the Rocky Mountains. Yes, I had two days where I couldn't participate, but enough to fill an album with family photographs of me in a very yellow jacket with so many zippers, the family would ask me to mind all their small things...like gloves, hats and energy bars. I was the mountain mule, in that regard!*

Q: *How was it possible to do balance sports with Meniere's?*

A: *If I felt even remotely dizzy I wouldn't do them. I waited for the right 'window'. I was core training and with a will to challenge myself, I found plenty of times for those sports I enjoyed. Being able to do things, keeps your mind off Meniere's.*

Q: *How did you utilize 'good days'?*

A: *As soon as I had a 'good day' even if it was just for* an hour or two, I would get up and get moving. I would challenge myself. If I began to feel unwell, I would stop the activity. I think I would have been a better skier and a better windsurfer if I were not attempting these sports under the shadow of Meniere's. I also think the instructors had the patience of saints because it took me twice if not three times longer to learn as I struggled with balance. But it was worth it in the end.

Q: *Was doing so many balance activities a conscious decision?*

A: *The remarkable thing is, I was drawn to balance activities on more of a subconscious level. It was after focusing on learning sports that required core strength and balance, that I read data about the benefits: the more balance activities you do during the first six months of a diagnosis, the better the prognosis. I had naturally gravitated to doing these balancing activities and I am sure doing that helped me in the long run to regain my equilibrium and recover.*

Q: *Did you take any risks when you had Meniere's?*

A: *Some were considered a little risky such as windsurfing, surfing, and snowboarding. Others such as core workouts weren't risky. Most of the risk was thinking it was all going to be too demanding. When you can't bend down and tie your shoelaces without feeling dizzy, it's hard to image doing almost any activity let alone demanding ones.*

ON THE QUESTION OF TRAVEL

Q: Why is getting out and about important?

A: Getting out and about allows you to be part of society and to feel normal. Not going out, puts sufferers at risk of isolation, loneliness, and depression.

Q: Did you ever have an attack while driving a car?

A: No. I never had an attack while driving a car. I took control of the car only when I felt capable. If your condition makes it difficult to operate a vehicle for a while, consider transportation alternatives such as public transport or getting out with a friend at the wheel.

Q: Did you plan your vacations or were they spontaneous?

A: Both. But even spontaneous vacations were planned in detail to avoid stress and fatigue.

Q: Can you go on a boat with Meniere's?

A: Yes, you can go on sailing ship, cruise ship or boat with an outboard. If you get seasick in rough weather, you won't be alone. Sailing won't give you a permanent feeling of wooziness. In fact, your balance system may well benefit from gentle rock and rolling because being at sea challenges your balance. I often went sailing and fishing in small craft while I had Meniere's. However, if I were having a series of bad days, then I wouldn't bother.

Q: Could you travel by train with Meniere's?

A: Yes, I could travel by train with Meniere's. A word of advice though for the journey; when looking out of the window, look into the far distance at objects, don't try and follow fast-moving images.

Q: How did you cope with air travel?

A: To help prevent fatigue, I avoided purchasing tickets on red-eye flights. I booked daytime flights; chose routes with the least time zone changes, and included stopovers where possible, to let my body catch up. The aim was not to get exhausted and travel fatigued. I'd booked an aisle seat away from service areas, in the forward section of the aircraft for better airflow. I would also book a seat over the wings, for less movement during turbulence. I used earplugs and eyes-hades to cut out light and noise, preorder low salt meals, stayed hydrated and avoided alcohol. Travel for me was about self-preservation on the outbound and inbound journey.

Q: *Did flying cause you ear pain?*

A: *I did long-haul plane trips and never once suffered ear pain. I was initially apprehensive thinking about how pressure would affect my Meniere's, but cabin pressure affects the middle ear, not the inner ear.*

Q: *What are your five important tips for travel?*

A: *Avoid getting overtired. Keep sight of your dietary requirements. Avoid stress. Make the most of your vacation time. Enjoy yourself!*

Q: *What was your most memorable travel experience?*

A: *Traveling with the family to the mountains and being Meniere free with no vertigo for two weeks. Comparatively, I always felt much better at altitude than I did at sea level!*

Q: *What was something you did that surprised you?*

A: *Arriving with family in Whistler, after a four-hour car journey from Vancouver. My Canadian friend, Al, handed out pairs of cross-country skis. It was 11:00pm on*

New Years Eve. If he had asked me beforehand, I would have said no, because I'd been feeling slightly 'off' the previous day. He had organized everything, so what could I say? So, we skied across icy wooden bridges and over snow covered fields; past stands of fir trees, in the moonlight. Quite a feat when I look back at it now. Proof you really can do more than you think you can, with Meniere's.

ON YOUR EXPERIENCE WITH MENIERE'S

Q: What happened in the months before you got Meniere's?

A: I had a four-month battle with a water-borne parasite I had contracted in the tropics. This required two courses of a very strong antiviral medicine. Shortly afterward, during an international trip for business, I had my first vertigo attack.

Q: How healthy or unhealthy were you when you got sick?

A: I had both healthy and unhealthy habits. I did gym regularly, was active in sports, walked and ate a healthy diet. But I also worked a sixty-hour week, socialized, drank copious cups of coffee and indulged in food and drink at regular late-night business occasions. Having a business and a young family occupied all my time. I was always on the go. I didn't take time out for myself as I considered myself healthy and capable. However, there were signs that I was on the verge of exhaustion. I ignored these and just accepted that was the way of it.

Q: *Did you blame your habits for making you sick?*

A: *If living a high stress dynamic busy life was my habit, well; yes it was one of my suspicions for why I was ill.*

Q: *Do you think you need to set boundaries for good health?*

A: *Most definitely yes. These boundaries also need to adapt to your age. One can have boundaries at 30 but those boundaries are no longer acceptable at 45. They need to be prioritized differently. Not necessarily reduced. Work smarter not harder.*

Q: *Describe your Meniere's disease onset?*

A: *Everyone seems to remember in detail the first attack of vertigo. I was in Paris on business. I was staying in a hotel opposite the Grand Opera House. However, no amount of opulent surroundings could rid me of the horrible spinning bout I was experiencing. I couldn't figure out what was causing me to feel so ill. I put it down to food poisoning from lunch I'd just eaten and called the hotel doctor. I realize now, it was the first vertigo attack.*

Q: How old were you when you were first diagnosed?

A: When I was diagnosed with Meniere's disease, I had just celebrated my 46th birthday.

Q: How did you feel about the age you were when diagnosed?

A: Forty-six years old was way too young to be diagnosed with an incurable disease.

Q: What was one of your most frightening moments?

A: Being in the early stages of an attack of vertigo and hearing a car alarm going off in the driveway. However, my wife told me there was no alarm outside or anywhere to be heard. This sound never left me. Later I learned it was the spontaneous onset of the roaring, ringing and blasting of Meniere's tinnitus.

Q: How do people react to a Meniere's diagnosis?

A: People diagnosed react in different ways, depending on their personalities. Some pretend it isn't happening or refuse to accept that they are ill; while others share the bad news and find comfort with family and friends.

Q: What did a Meniere's disease diagnosis mean to you?

A: It was incomprehensible to me. Not part of my life

plan. Having an unexpected, confrontational, unpredictable, distressing and challenging disease to deal with, left me in a state of numbness. It left me in confusion. It was a disease that had no boundaries and no rhyme or reason. I had no definitive course of action to deal with it.

Q: *How did you feel when you were diagnosed?*

A: *I think it was one of the worst days of my life. I wasn't really expecting to be diagnosed with anything. I just thought I had an ear infection. I didn't understand why I had Meniere's. I was a seemingly fit man, at the height of my professional career, running my own business. I was a founding executive owner of this company. Married with a young family of two, one in primary school and one child at intermediate school. Over fifty people directly relied on me at work, plus my entire family. I couldn't afford to be sick.*

Q: *How would you sum up your diagnosis, in five words?*

A: *Confusion. Shock. Fear. Loss. Trepidation.*

Q: *Did a Meniere's diagnosis leave you with regret, shame or guilt?*

A: *Yes, all three. Regret that I hadn't taken more care of myself. Guilt about not being able to control and stabilize my home and financial life. Shame about having, what I considered a weakness, a disease. Such feelings of despair are a* *breeding ground for negative thoughts.*

Q: Was there ever a time when your blood ran cold?

A: It had to be when the doctor slapped on that label of an incurable chronic condition called Meniere's. I thought I was truly doomed.

Q: What comes to mind when you hear the word vertigo?

A: The way Meniere vertigo takes you into the vortex of a spinning hyperspace.

Q: What was your prognosis for Meniere disease?

A: The ENT specialist told me I would have Meniere's for life. He added that there was no cure for it. I was given no real answers about Meniere's disease. It was extremely difficult to know what to do or how to cope. It was all too clear the patterns of my life were about to be shattered. It was very unclear what lay ahead for me and my family. What I didn't understand at the time was this. While there is no one cure for Meniere's, that didn't mean I could never get better. But I took 'no cure' as meaning: I was always going to have vertigo attacks.

Q: On a scale of one to ten how sad did Meniere's make you feel?

A: One. I was extremely upset about the fact that my

life was revolving around Meniere attacks. I would wake up thinking about Meniere's, spend the day thinking about Meniere's and go to sleep worrying about Meniere's. It wasn't like anything I had encountered before; like a bad flu when after a couple of weeks you recover. It was all consuming initially until I put my self-help regime in place and gained control.

Q: *What was your idea of a bad day with Meniere's?*

A: *A vertigo attack with associated vomiting.*

Q: *Did you get warning signs for an attack?*

A: *Yes. I would feel strangely exhausted, a feeling of being dog tired even if I hadn't been doing much to warrant that kind of tiredness. At the same time, my hearing would drop and I would have trouble hearing what people were saying; a sensation of cotton wool compacted in my ears made sound quite muffled. Tinnitus picked up and seemed louder. Wooziness increased.*

Q: *When you had a vertigo attack, how would you do?*

A: *I would lie on my back, without moving my head a millimeter. Any movement to left or right increased the spinning dramatically.*

Q: *What did you think about most when you were lying in bed?*

A: When I moved, would I feel dizzy or normal? I had real difficulty trying not to think worrying thoughts. I tried to relax, let responsibilities go for the time being. I found the best thought was nothing.

Q: What is the most embarrassing thing that happened?

A: In the first months after diagnosis; having an attack and vomiting the meal I'd just eaten into a trashcan outside the Lebanese restaurant, and then staggering around the pavement in full view of restaurant patrons who had watched the entire scene unfold.

Q: What was one vertigo episode that lasted too long?

A: We were on holiday for a week and I had one bout of vertigo after another. I called them cluster attacks. Meniere's followed me on that vacation.

Q: How did you typically react in an acute attack?

A: I lay quietly and knew I had to ride out vertigo. I retained the thought, this will end soon. I will get better.

Q: On a scale of 1-10 how bad is a vertigo attack?

A: Zero. The worst feeling possible.

Q: How intense can vertigo attacks be?

A: Extremely intense. There is no other experience I

have had that compares with the awful sensation. Rotational spinning for an hour, is something non-sufferers could never begin to understand.

Q: How many days did your worst bouts of vertigo last?

A: I recorded a series of 12 attacks over a month.

Q: How often did you get vertigo?

A: The first year was the worst. I experienced attacks three or four times a month roughly.

Q: Did you ever go to the emergency room?

A: No. Luckily the doctor did house calls and twice he came and administered a shot to help the acute episode.

Q: Who gave you the most support?

A: My wife.

Q: In an emergency whom did you call?

A: I would call for my wife. She really understood my plight. She also planned, organized, researched and did a lot to make my time with Meniere's less complicated.

Q: Did Meniere's give you panic attacks?

A: Yes. At the slightest sensation of dizziness, I'd have flashes of anxiety. My heart would race and I'd break out

168

in the cold sweat of a panic attack. It was a vicious circle because high anxiety intensifies vertigo.

Q: Meniere's brings uncertainty. How did you cope ?

A: Meniere's certainly brings uncertainty. As well as trying to cope with vertigo attacks, the loss of life's equilibrium gave me an increasing worry about where Meniere's disease was taking my family, and me as well. But there was a feeling I have always had, that there is a light at the end of the tunnel. Often when I meditated, I tried to see or feel the light at the end of the tunnel and work my way towards it. It's hard to explain what that is exactly. A faith or a hope for a better outcome, but I always felt myself going towards a solution with all of this. I also instigated a management plan for coping with Meniere's with the end objective of getting better. All of this helped with the uncertainty.

Q: Did Meniere's affect your sense of well-being?

A: Yes, definitely. For the first time in my life, I felt a constant sense of anxiety and fear, which sapped my physical energy. The specialists couldn't give me definitive answers on how to manage the condition. Not knowing what to do made things worse for my sense of well-being for sure.

Q: What mood were you usually in?

A: In the early days, I was in a preoccupied rather indecisive state, all due to the uncertainty of vertigo attacks.

Q: Did Meniere's make you feel alone?

A: Often very alone. Support groups were non-existent. Had there been support groups, I would have had an easier time coping at the onset of the disease.

Q: Did you ever feel like a slave to Meniere's disease?

A: In the beginning, Meniere's certainly ruled my life. But the more I understood the triggers and how I was feeling, the more in control I felt. I was able to predict an oncoming attack and back things off; so the attacks became less frequent and not as violent. Understanding the mechanism of the vertigo attack really helped. I was able to apply a management plan to the vertigo attack with what I call the B.M.E. I was able to apply these to the Beginning, Middle, and End of the attack. It made a tremendous difference to being in control of the most disruptive symptom of Meniere's.

Q: What were the 'lows' of Meniere's?

A: Definitely the acute attacks of vertigo. For a long while, I felt like they were breaking my spirit, until I began to understand the components of attacks. Only then could I work towards reducing and eliminating them.

Q: *What did you do when you felt overburdened?*

A: *A common cause of stress is having too much to do and too little time in which to do it. I accepted I couldn't complete tasks if I felt overburdened. What was interesting was this. I found that really nothing needed to be completed today. Tomorrow or sometimes never, was OK too.*

Q: *Did confrontation with others affect you?*

A: *Most definitely. The confrontation aspect with people was one of the worst things, for me. Emotional blowouts, by their stressful nature, can put you in the vertigo attack zone. I learned to pick my battles and not sweat as much small stuff. To let things be.*

Q: *Could you argue with your wife?*

A: *A personal question! I could argue in small doses only. Not that I ever liked to resolve issues by arguing. I made every effort to avoid conflict, however, this, as you know, isn't always possible. I also think partner's need to cut Meniere sufferers some slack and avoid getting into conflicts to spare the Meniere sufferer the consequences.*

Q: *How did you keep the peace?*

A: *I tried not to sweat the small stuff. In fact, I read the book, 'Don't Sweat The Small Stuff' by Richard Carlson. Arguments were never worth the stress at the time and the*

*fallout afterward. I also meditated. I attempted to be more
positive and try to see the bigger picture. Meniere's made me
a little micro-focused. I used to be a big picture guy but small
things started to get to me.*

*Q: When you found yourself in a stressful situation, what
did you do?*

*A: Sometimes, I would stay and settle it. Most times I
would have to walk away. I advocate walking away to talk
another day, gives each person time to think. Then both people
can add some intelligence to the situation.*

Q: Did arguments cause Meniere vertigo attacks?

*A: I can't say for sure, but after an argument, I would
invariably have an attack in the days following. I really
advocate avoiding stress.*

Q: Did you feel angry at times?

*A: I am sure I became more prone to mild anger
outbursts. The anger outbursts were mainly due to
frustration.*

Q: How did you deal with anger?

*A: Striving toward a goal was my antidote to anger.
This basic rule was my key to dealing with anger.*

Q: *What things made you feel depressed sometimes?*

A: *Not being able to achieve what I used to achieve. I had a dreadful feeling of uncertainty about the future.*

Q: *Did you secretly long to be rescued?*

A: *I wanted a mentor for Meniere's. To talk to someone who had been through what I was going through; to show me where the pitfalls and hopefully where opportunities were; to give me life guidelines in a time of confusion.*

Q: *What was missing in your life with Meniere's?*

A: *Optimum health and the freedom to do exactly what I wanted to do without having to factor Meniere's into the living equation.*

Q: *What part of Meniere's had the biggest impact on you?*

A: *The feeling of uncertainty, of not knowing where Meniere's would take me. Not being totally independent.*

Q: *What fears did you have to overcome?*

A: *I had to get over the fear of not knowing when the next vertigo attack would happen. The fear of never getting a strong positive life back.*

Q: *What are things you never shared with anyone?*

A: Not to be able to function at 100%. I hated that feeling. And not being in control of my life, while everyone around me was moving on with theirs as normal.

Q: Did you ever seek counseling?

A: I did. I felt such an overwhelming personal struggle with the loss of career and health at the same time. Unchecked grief, guilt, and shame made me begin to feel worthless, inadequate and insignificant. I really had to do something. I had a very supportive psychologist whom I would see, not on a regular basis, but whenever I felt overwhelmed by Meniere's and the associated issues it brought to me. My psychologist was a specialist in post-traumatic disorder PTD and had suffered a major trauma himself in his previous career. He helped me cope with loss and grief.

Q: What questions did you ask yourself?

A: How do I make a new life with the condition? Can I get better? Will I be able to work dynamically again? Will my relationships completely change now? Will we lose our financial position? How do we survive?

Q: Do you think there is a certain amount of denial?

A: If you're in denial, you're trying to protect yourself by refusing to accept the truth about something that's happening in your life. To some degree, initial short-term denial can be a good thing. It can give time to adjust to a stressful issue. It can also give you time to look at the possibility for a life change. But denial has a dark side. Being in denial for too long can prevent you from dealing with issues that require action, such as a financial situation - it can be a roadblock.

Q: *Did you live in denial at all?*

A: *For sure. As an active, physical man, I found the diagnosis almost impossible to accept. I saw it as a weakness at 46. I was embarrassed to admit that I now had a permanent condition. I tried to pretend to everyone I was normal, nothing wrong. I didn't want to 'identity' with Meniere's. Then I thought things like...the specialist is wrong, I don't have Meniere's. I wasn't fooling myself. As well as the denial, I was concerned about how Meniere's was going to impact my life and how we'd live with the fallout.*

Q: *Did denial make things better or worse?*

A: *For me, denial only made things worse. I kept trying to do things at my usual pace and under the same pressures, but it made the attacks worse.*

Q: *How long were you in denial?*

A: *At least three months! I tried to ignore the fact that Meniere's was going to change my life significantly. I kept going with my habits of drinking coffee and working long* *hours. But as symptoms got worse, Meniere's demanded I altered habits of a lifetime.*

Q: How long until you accepted you had Meniere's?

A: I began to adapt to Meniere's being part of my life. That point was the beginning of my journey towards getting better. Every ending creates a new beginning, as long as you know when one journey ends and the other begins.

ON THE QUESTION OF GETTING BETTER

Q: *What motivated you towards recovery?*

A: *I'd had a week of vertigo attacks. When I managed to get myself up, I went and sat for a long time in the garden under the proverbial old apple tree, with its rope swing for the kids; the tree was in need of a prune and a spray, its trunk covered with lichen, yet it was full of apple blossom, with bees buzzing. My young daughter came home from school and asked me to push her on the swing. I found the simple act of anticipating the rise and fall of the swing very demanding. I realized that even the simple tasks of normal life were almost beyond me. It was a kind of self-motivation that kicked in from then on. I decided to take responsibility for figuring out how to overcome this debilitating condition. I refused to be the sick Dad. And I was learning windsurfing and skiing with her in a matter of months.*

Q: Who encouraged you to make a full recovery?

A: I encouraged myself to make strategies and set goals I could achieve. My family was always there to support me.

Q: Why was accepting your condition important to you?

A: Accepting having Meniere's was part of the cure. I no longer berated myself, instead I decided to embrace a healthy coexistence with Meniere's. For me, accepting the condition came from figuring out the possible causes, for why I had the condition. Then I found ways to live with it. Once I'd found ways to live with the disease, I found ways to beat it.

Q: When did you decide to not wallow in Meniere's disease?

A: I was never a guy who would give in easily. Quite early on in my diagnosis, I thought about the prognosis the doctor had given me. When someone says you will have the disease for life and there is little you can do about it, just made me feel like it was the end of my life. I had heard of people who have suffered Meniere's disease for decades. The swing with my daughter was the turning point that snapped me out of the Meniere doldrums.

Q: Did you develop a personal philosophy?

A: My personal philosophy was more of a mantra: 'I will get better'. I took responsibility for my health.

Q: How did you go about recovering?

A: To be honest, when you feel really bad and are suffering with symptoms, it is hard to find any space to do anything. It all seems too difficult. I had to start somewhere because there was no way I could wait until I felt better. Meniere symptoms were there most days. So I began by taking every opportunity I could, no matter how small it seemed or how insignificant, I would do one thing towards recovery. I started a simple achievable self-help management plan to improve my health; including meditation, diet, walking, and supplements. I also understood that it wasn't a single plan, it had to be a stepping stone approach. Achieve one goal and step to the next goal.

Q: What was the best thing you did towards a recovery?

A: The month I began to walk first two lamp-posts then four, then around the block. A very simple act, but it put me in control. The more I achieved in health, the more I was able to cope with Meniere's.

Q: What do you think made a difference?

A: I believe it wasn't one thing, but every little thing I did, that made a difference. Small details are easy to overlook:

like writing in a diary, avoiding salt, meditating, going for a walk, appreciating nature, learning a new skill...doing these small things every day, worked for me.

Q: *Was getting better an easy thing to do?*

A: *No. It wasn't easy or fast but doable and achievable with a modicum of what I call the "Three P's": patience, perseverance and persistence.*

Q: *If you were to sum up your philosophy for recovery?*

A: *Common sense. I'd say making a recovery involved doing a lot of seemingly basic and simple things. We tend to overlook the most basic things these days, for example: resting, and enjoying nature. Nowadays we can pop a tablet to calm down or sleep, disguise a headache or flu, all so we can soldier on. But at what cost to overall health? The self-help techniques I figured out were simple enough to apply every day. They worked to eventually eliminate Meniere's.*

Q: *What are five things for someone just diagnosed?*

A: *Firstly, accept the condition. It's not easy, but once you acknowledge the disease, you can begin to manage your health. Secondly, is to have a belief in yourself that you can and will get better. Keep fanning a flame of hope in your mind. Thirdly, because you are the one who needs to make a recovery, accept responsibility for getting better. Fourthly,* *adopt a very positive attitude and keep as many aspects of your life positive. Fifthly, gain information about Meniere's because knowledge is key. Spend as much time learning about Meniere's, as you spend worrying about it. There are now books, websites, support groups and societies, medical sites and public libraries to help you learn about Meniere's.*

Q: *What were the resolutions you made?*

A: *Not to get lost in the symptoms of the disease and realize the symptoms were not who I was, it was Meniere's. Not to let Meniere's define me as a person. To believe that if I could reduce and eliminate the symptoms, I would get my life back; which turned out to be true.*

Q: *What was your personal strategy?*

A: *At first, I monitored my everyday activities to establish what was aggravating Meniere's symptoms. Then I developed self-help strategies and worked on changing what I thought the issues were.*

Q: *Name the five most significant purchases you made?*

A: *The monthly membership at the local gum. Cross-training shoes for walking and doing gym. Noise blocker for noise recruitment. A low-salt cookbook. Windsurfers for my daughter and myself.*

Q: *How did you exercise your mind?*

A: Reading books, listening to music, watching documentaries, spending time in the kitchen, travel, painting, and writing. Learning new activities.

Q: Did you become more laid-back, or more intense?

A: Laid-back was not my personality, but when I suffered Meniere symptoms, I was forced onto my back. Now people say I am a more laid back. I think that's good!

Q: How many hours did you work on the computer?

A: I only spent time at computers in film post-production sessions. Computers were not a big part of my day-to-day work. When I decided to learn computer programs in the early stages of Meniere's, I suffered from attacks after sitting down at the computer for twenty minutes or so. I kept away from using computers, for the first year.

Q: How long was it before you could spend time on the computer?

A: After eighteen months, I managed fifteen minutes and then gradually worked my way up to half an hour. Now I have recovered, I can spend most of the day on the computer. However, I always take proper breaks from the screen. I no longer work as hard-out as I did in the past.

Q: What effect did the computer have?

A: The brightness of the screen and the vertical scrolling movement was enough to trigger a Meniere's attack. I also found the computer made me tired.

Q: What do you say to people with Meniere's?

A: I meet a lot of sufferers who have continual acute vertigo attacks. Between attacks they post (on the computer) about how bad the attacks were! Honestly, if you are having umpteen vertigo attacks, and wonder why you have them... take a hard look at how much time you're spending on the computer, without taking proper breaks.

Q: Why have you not written this book as an e-book?

A: The people I want to reach with this 'Q & A' book are the newly diagnosed, or those who are so disabled by symptoms, they can't spend hours on the computer.

Q: How long could you spend reading a book?

A: Initially, I could only read for twenty minutes to half an hour at a time. Activities involving eye movements were problematic at the start.

Q: And if you had to choose one book for sufferers?

A: No question about this recommendation here. 'I read the following book cover to cover. 'Full Catastrophe Living', a book based on Jon Kabat-Zinn's renowned mindfulness-

based stress reduction program. It helped me with day to day stress. 'Full Catastrophe Living' taught me mindfulness which helped me with health and healing. The book is a positive game-changer.

Q: Did you read any other of his books?

A: Yes. I read 'Wherever You Go, There You Are', first published in 1994.

Q: How did you plan for a good night's sleep?

A: A lack of sleep is a significant cause of stress. I would spend time relaxing before going to sleep and stop doing any mentally demanding tasks four hours before going to bed. I often had a warm bath, read a lightweight book, just enough to allow my brain to calm down.

Q: When sleeping, did you keep your head flat or raised?

A: I always used a couple of pillows.

Q: When you slept, did you prefer to be flat on your back?

A: I preferred to sleep on my side.

Q: What position did you usually wake up in?

A: Exactly the same position.

Q: Did you count sheep if you had trouble sleeping?

A: No, definitely not. I'd get out of bed, and eat a banana for the potassium. I found lying in bed not sleeping, created anxiety.

Q: When was it impossible to sleep?

A: I'd lie on the sofa looking at the lights of the city and the infinity of stars, the light of all helps to create a greater perspective, in a universal sense, I think.

Q: Did it help to have animals around?

A: I like animals around and find them a comfort. But definitely not in the bed. We used to have our three cats sleep on the bed, but I found they would wake me up. So the family pets had to find somewhere else to sleep.

Q: Did you feel you got enough sleep?

A: Yes, although I was always tired with the condition.

Q: What time would you wake up in the mornings?

A: Usually, I would wake up twice. In the early hours before the sparrows woke, I would be aware of how I was feeling. If things felt normal I would go back to sleep and wake again about 8 am.

Q: Were mornings your worst time of day?

A: No, those tended to be the late afternoons. During the *night, if I woke with a vertigo attack, the morning was a recovery time.*

Q: *What did you do when you got out of bed?*

A: *I got out of bed around 8 pm. As soon as I was awake, I would have breakfast. I needed to fuel up as soon as possible after waking.*

Q: *What was your favorite place in the house?*

A: *The back veranda overlooking the garden. The arbor drooping with clusters of purple wisteria, in the heat of summer.*

Q: *Did you take rests during the day?*

A: *I certainly did. I planned a rest mid-morning and then mid-afternoon. This was my time for meditation, as well as taking time out for myself.*

Q: *What do you recommend for meditation?*

A: *The four-part home training course, Jon Kabat-Zinn offers. His mindfulness meditation practice on CD gave me very deep states of relaxation and sense of well-being.*

Q: *Did your thoughts drift off places during meditation?*

A: *Focus is meditation and I found focus the most beneficial. When I used guided meditations, I would often* select water themes. I was brought up as a happy kid on the beach. So yes, the ocean was my drift.

Q: *What made you decide to produce a meditation CD?*

A: *When I suffered from Meniere symptoms, I regularly listened to a series of guided meditations. I borrowed these from the local library and I listened to a meditation audio at least once a day. Some were guided meditations with a spoken voice, directing the flow of meditation. I also listened to ocean waves as a meditation. I was inspired by Jon Kabat-Zinn and thought it may help others to hear a guided meditation by a person who had Meniere's.*

Q: *Describe your "Epic Nap"?*

A: *The 90-minute epic nap is one complete sleep cycle. Initially, it proved difficult to stay conscious during an entire 60-minute meditation. Somewhere along the way, I would drift off and have one of my epic naps. When I woke up, the meditation had well and truly finished.*

Q: *Tell us about the "Power Nap"?*

A: *My power nap was a sleep session that happened during the day (ideally between 1:00 to 4:00 pm), which lasted between 10 and 30 minutes. This I found essential to maintain energy and to give me a sense of refreshment.*

Q: *What was your "Refresher Nap"?*

A: I would take a refresher nap after and often before an activity. I could nap 20 minutes exactly and feel refreshed. Any longer and I ran the risk of "sleep inertia" — that unpleasant groggy feeling that takes a long time to shake off. I avoided naps later than 4:00 pm because I found it disrupted regular sleep.

Q: If you spent one hour doing nothing, what did you do?

A: I'd sit in the sunshine overlooking the bay. I always found it relaxing to sit and observe the boats, bird-life, sunsets, clouds and weather patterns.

Q: What paradox in life have you had to learn or accept?

A: Laziness! Laziness is nothing more than the habit of resting before you get tired. Laziness works. It's a way of incorporate health benefits into your life. I always thought laziness was a bad habit but now I don't, preferring to take a 'laissez-faire' attitude; which simply means "let go" or "let them do it" or "leave it to itself", while you rest mind and body. It also helps with that busy attitude of; I must get everything done now. With Meniere's, this is not the right attitude. Far better to let 'invisible hands' do the work for you, while you take a break.

Q: Did Meniere's make you a creature of habit?

A: I have always been a creature of habit. I gave up a

few bad habits such as working late at night on the computer and adopted healthy habits, like walking every day. I put more routine into my life. I noticed it took four months to get into a habit, such as going to the gym on a regular basis. It also took four months to break a bad habit and replace it with something healthy; like swapping caffeinated coffee for a hot lemon and honey drink. I found it easy to slip back into old patterns until the 4 month timeframe.

Q: *Did Meniere's create any idiosyncrasies?*

A: *In the early stages of Meniere's, I made a definite decision. I would beat this disease and get well. If I was going to get back to normal, I knew I would have to figure this Meniere thing out on my own. This created some idiosyncrasies because, for the first time in my life, I had to focus on my self, 'self-monitor' my activities to see the connection between 'triggers' and what I was doing. Self-help does put emphasis on the self. I had to put myself first, and that was a new paradigm for me.*

Q: *Did you plan your day or did the day plan you?*

A: *If I didn't wake with acute vertigo symptoms, I would plan my day by making a list. I tried to not stack things one on top of the other but pace myself. If I didn't do what I wanted in a day, I would shift it to the following day. I became better at personal time management. Running myself on full power was no longer part of my agenda.*

Q: *How important was it to set goals?*

A: *Goal setting is paramount. Belief can also act as a goal. I believe in the quantum physics of belief. You have to believe you will get better.*

Q: *Why is learning to say "No" so important?*

A: *Learning to say "No" helped to reduce my level of stress. I stopped taking on additional responsibility. I practiced saying phrases such as: "I am sorry but I can't commit to this at the moment." "Now is not a good time as I'm in the middle of something. "Why don't you ask me again at..." "Maybe later." "I'll let you know..." "Let me give that some thought." "I'd love to do this, but ...". If you are used to being the "Yes" person, you might have to take a step back. There are only so many hours in the day —taking time for yourself is essential for reducing symptoms.*

Q: *When you were feeling unwell, did you keep on going?*

A: *No I didn't carry on regardless. I would take a rest. Often this simple act diverted a vertigo attack. When you are feeling well, you still must stop and rest.*

Q: *What did you consider a good day with Meniere's?*

A: *If I did everything in the day with my self-help management plan, such as exercise, do everything on my list without feeling bad or exhausted.*

Q: *What did you consider a really good day?*

A: *Feeling relaxed, doing everything I wanted to do and having a normal day without any sign of Meniere's. These were my 'windows' where I felt I was living my life to the full again. Sometimes these great days were followed by a bad day, but the more self-help I did, the more really good days I seemed to have. I really felt I was on the mend.*

Q: *How did you react when you finally 'managed' your attacks?*

A: *It was an amazing feeling. I sat down and worked out what I call the B.M.E, The Beginning, Middle and End of attacks. Then, through applying simple measures at each of the stages, the attacks became less intense, less frequent, less frightening. The space between attacks became longer and then no attacks at all. It took time but I started to feel more and more confident and I was going have a future. Every day, since my recovery, I feel thankful.*

Q: *What lesson did Meniere's make you learn the hard way?*

A: *If I didn't take notice of when I was tired or stressed, I would have a vertigo attack. The consequence of not taking care was ruthless. To counter this, I listened to my body more and stopped going into exhaustion mode. As soon as I felt tired or stressed, I would take a break. Gradually my energy levels* *increased, because I didn't run myself down and drain my energy reserves.*

Q: What stressed you out most?

A: Initially, day to day demands and not being able to meet them.

Q: What advice can you give to relieve stress?

A: Avoid stressful situations and activities, especially the consumption of nicotine and any drinks containing caffeine and alcohol. All of these are stimulants that increase levels of stress and tinnitus. Stress increases the level of stress hormones. Walking and other kinds of physical activity help to metabolize excess stress hormones. This helps the body and mind calm down. When I felt stressed or tense, I'd go for a walk in fresh air and literally step into a more relaxed state.

Q: What other ideas can you share for relieving stress?

A: Just talking to someone about how you're feeling can help. Talking helps in two ways. Chatting about things can distract you from stressful thoughts. Discussing problems can help release built-up tension caused by stressful issues. Spend time in nature.

Q: What did you do when you needed to relax?

A: *I'd soak for a long time in a warm bath with aromatherapy oils.*

Q: Did you often feel overwhelmed?

A: Yes. In the initial months.

Q: What did you do to 'get centered'?

A: I focused on small activities that were achievable. This gave me a sense of success and momentum.

Q: What made you feel OK?

A: Simple things really. A cup of decaffeinated coffee; reading the morning paper at a café down the road. Or the occasional fish and chips (without salt) wrapped in newspaper, sitting in the park down by the wharf building. The same wharf I jumped off as a boy. It was nice just being able to do simple things and get out and about. Later I loved windsurfing in a sea estuary, listening to the gulls on a beautiful blue water day, with my daughter who loved doing things with her dad.

Q: Did Meniere's make you superstitious?

A: Not superstitious but vigilant. Once I set myself a goal to get better, it wasn't easy. I was constantly monitoring myself: food, supplements, and activities. I was very aware of how I was feeling so I could adjust things accordingly. Some things may have looked a little superstitious like looking at the clouds building up and saying, this could be trouble, because the barometric pressure was a trigger for me.

Q: *Did you believe you would ever get better?*

A: *I was told at the onset, I would always have Meniere's. When I was having acute Meniere's attacks, I couldn't look up normally without going dizzy. I couldn't tie my shoelaces without feeling woozy. At the time, I never imagined I would get back to normal; I really did wonder if I would ever make a recovery or if Meniere's was the new normal for me. Some days I felt really hopeless. I couldn't believe this was happening to me. Worse, I had no idea what to do about the relentless attacks of vertigo I was suffering. There seemed to be no end to it. Some days were also better than others, but these were few and far between. I lived each day in constant fear of the next vertigo attack. It was only when I started to manage Meniere's and gain some control, that this sense of hopelessness changed for the better. I am also sure that having a strong belief is the best medicine. Believing you can recover from Meniere's is paramount. Just keep a recovery in your mind. Never waiver from it, no matter what. Bad days with Meniere's will always test your strength. Keep believing you can and will get better. Even if you don't believe it when things feel really bad, just fake it to start with! Beliefs do grow over time. The more you believe, the more it will come through. Belief accompanied by actions* is a very powerful law of nature for success.

Q: *Did you lose faith at all?*

A: *Yes. During weeks of constant vertigo, I really did lose both faith and hope. Around that time, simple contact with nature, having close family around, and even the pet cats seemed to help get me through. I took notice of the small things and appreciated the little things more.*

Q: *To what extent will a person's attitude influence healing?*

A: *It takes the right attitude, a positive one, and a belief that you can figure out how to reduce acute symptoms, increase health and wellness. You can change your attitude like the flick of an 'ON' switch. I really do believe in the quantum physics of healing. Meniere's is a disease that your body has at the moment. This can make you feel that your life has been taken over by the condition. You would never choose Meniere's in a million years, but you have the ability to influence the direction your life will take. In order to make permanent change, you have to look at all aspects of your life. It is possible to do the seemingly impossible.*

Q: *What's something you lost through having Meniere's?*

A: *The career I had built up and all that goes with years of hard work.*

Q: What is something you found through Meniere's?

A: I found that I listened to my body. I was more aware of actions and reactions. How one thing affects another. This self-awareness acted as a map back to a personal sense of inherent well-being.

Q: What is the worst thing a non-Meniere sufferer said?

A: "Meniere's is a mere minor inconvenience."

Q: What drove you crazy about Meniere's?

A: Not being in control. It created an unnerving feeling. Not being able to find answers seemed to exasperate how I felt. When I regularly experienced spontaneous vertigo, I lost confidence in the stability of my life.

Q: What has been the biggest challenge of Meniere's?

A: Not allowing Meniere's disease to take over my life and personality but to work with it, to beat the symptoms. Getting that balance right helped me look after myself and yet, move ahead towards recovery.

Q: What was your greatest life challenge?

A: Losing a successful career to Meniere's and re-figuring my life from there.

Q: What was your strongest attribute for recovery?

A: A positive attitude. In times of serious illness, you must hold a strong belief in a positive outcome, regardless of the hell you are going through at the time. It takes a positive attitude to keep a positive outlook. Positivity overall is what gives one the strength to overcome the disabling effects of Meniere's disease. A positive attitude is a powerful medicine.

Q: What was something Meniere's changed about you?

A: My sense of certainty changed. I tend to not project my future so far out. I have a three-month plan and a six-month plan. I live more in the present than the past or the future. I increased my sense of self-preservation and look after myself more.

Q: What could Meniere's never change about you?

A: My positive attitude, sense of humor, zest for living, never underestimate the power of love and strength of family ties. I always had a 'sort this mess out' attitude. A belief in self-determination.

Q: What do you never take for granted?

A: Appreciating good health these days. I feel more than lucky. I feel privileged to have a second chance at doing life.

Q: What did you do in your free time?

A: This changed as the disease progressed and I

improved in health. But initially the list would be; sit on the sofa, rest, sit outside, walk, rest, even go shopping. Then later many things were home-based like doing fix-up jobs around the house, renovating, cooking, barbecue, working in the garden, reading, watching TV, listening to music, doing gym, walking, being a family guy. Then, I was able to add in more sports activities and go out in a boat, go fishing, and go traveling. After my recovery, I was able to do everything I did before, except scuba diving.

Q: What should you never feel guilty about?

A: Feeling lazy, taking breaks and taking time out.

Q: Did Meniere's make you serious minded?

A: No. They say laughter is the best medicine. Even on the worst days, I kept my humor.

Q: How can humor help with Meniere's?

A: When you are down, switch to the comedy channel, and watch funny programs. A good laugh goes a long way to having a happy life.

Q: What was something that brought a smile to your face?

A: Comedy. I spent time watching laugh-out-loud comedy programs. I think it helped change my perspective and lighten up. Humor, whether an in-house joke or seeing the funny side, picked me up whenever I was feeling down.

Q: *Do you believe positivity helped in your recovery?*

A: *Yes. Once I was over the initial shock. I worked on maintaining a positive attitude by taking every effort to replace negative thoughts with positive ones.*

Q: *Did you watch movies?*

A: *Yes, I did, but I learned by trial, and error, never to sit anywhere in the front rows. I'd pick seats in the middle, or back of a movie theatre, with the screen directly in front of me. Although I'm a die-hard movie buff, I walked out halfway through movies like 'Breaking Waves' because of its vigorous hand-held camera-work. I had to walk out of films that went in and out of focus with jumps cuts and high action scenes. You can find lists of vertigo-inducing movies on the Internet, for example, 'The Walk', where shots are panning up as well as looking down. Films in 3D add visual complications because the eye's natural focal point is tricked to create the visual effects.*

Q: *What is your favorite Meniere Man quote?*

A: *The more you do...the more you can do.*

Q: *Where was your favorite place to be?*

A: At home. The home was a sanctuary for me on so many levels.

Q: What was your favorite season?

A: The summer season because the barometric levels were more settled.

Q: Do you think hot or cold weather affects symptoms the most?

A: Winter for sure. Not so much the cold, but storms and unsettled weather. I was affected by barometric pressure, the weather patterns of low-pressure fronts. Then there was the flu and lack of vitamin D.

Q: What one thing did you wish for most?

A: Good health. To put Meniere's disease behind me.

Q: What t-shirt slogan would you write for Meniere's disease?

A: Breathe.

Q: Which of your five senses do you treasure the most?

A: I treasure the sense of hearing. The Otosclerosis in my unaffected ear (from surfing in cold water) has progressed to nearly completely blocking the hearing in my left ear. Missing out on communication, birds... pretty well everything, it's a really big loss.

Q: *And if you were forced to give up one of your senses?*

A: *You do realize when you lose an aspect of your senses, how important they are to feeling alive. I don't want to give up any more senses.*

Q: *What's something you regret losing most?*

A: *I regret losing the things I can never find again, like my hearing, I will never get that back again.*

Q: *What are the best sounds to your ears?*

A: *Birdsong, chirping crickets at night, and the ocean waves.*

Q: *What are the worst sounds?*

A: *Loud sharp noises like firecrackers; sudden noise and someone talking to me very quietly.*

Q: *Did you listen to music or prefer quiet?*

A: *I preferred quiet when I suffered from Meniere's.*

Q: *What are the lasting legacies of having had Meniere's?*

A: *Roaring tinnitus and deafness in the affected ear.*

Q: *What was your greatest achievement with Meniere's?*

A: Doing normal activities without having a Meniere's attack. Succeeding at sports or social events without having an attack. Normality is a big achievement.

Q: What events brought about the greatest life-changes?

A: Having children and being responsible for their care and upbringing. That changed me into a family man. And being diagnosed with Meniere's because that altered my career path.

Q: And when people don't understand Meniere?

A: It depends on who it is and what effect they have on you. I know one man who had all the information on the condition, and had an elderly mother who suffered with Meniere's, yet he still referred to Meniere's as a mere minor inconvenience; to me, that defies credibility and shows a total lack of empathy.

Q: What issues about Meniere's fire you up?

A: Lack of understanding by non-sufferers. Yes, even family and friends can be dismissive and expect one to just get over it, which is truly demeaning. Sufferers are vulnerable on a physical, mental, and emotional level because they don't often receive the support necessary to cope. And worse, people who have Meniere's disease may be taken advantage of. The fact is, there are people in society who are aggressive predators looking to take advantage. These people exist. So be aware and seek as much genuine support as you can.

Q: What one thing is detrimental to recovery?

A: Don't swallow the bitter pill! Harboring grudges, petty jealousies, stressing about everything, holding a negative attitude towards life and how life is treating you. Try to avoid the negative: whether a thought, word, or deed. Every negative action has a reaction. Switch the negative off. It's easy to let Meniere's get you down, to adopt a negative focus and live a Meniere's life, as your new way of life. I advocate doing the complete opposite. Adopt a positive attitude. In my experience, the more you let go of negativity, the more Meniere's lets go of you.

Q: What do you recommend to overcome self-pity?

A: "Act and act now."

Q: What would have been a game-changer for you?

A: To have had comprehensive information about Meniere's, when I was diagnosed.

Q: If you could have eliminated one limitation?

A: The vertigo attacks because they were the most debilitating aspect of the condition. Many things in life seem beyond our control at first.

Q: *If you had been assured you would get better?*

A: *I would have attempted to keep my career going by taking a long leave of absence and coming back to work as I could manage. I wouldn't have given up my position in the company. Extreme problems require careful solutions.*

Q: *If you could change one thing, what would that be?*

A: *That I had been diagnosed this year, when a lot more information and research is available to sufferers.*

Q: *If you could give a gift to a sufferer?*

A: *The gift of a complete recovery.*

Q: *If you could cure a disease what would it be?*

A: *Alzheimer's disease.*

Q: *What potent advice would you give to sufferers?*

A: *The more you do, the better you feel. The better you feel, the more you achieve.*

Q: *If you had Meniere's now, what would you do?*

A: *I would seek as much advice as possible before I made any major decisions.*

Q: *Was your illness part of life?*

A: I would say Meniere's was like a season, the winter of my life. Initially, I was faced with a very bleak outlook. I would say the initial first stage of Meniere's were the worst years for everyone in my family.

Q: What residual reminders do you have?

A: Physically these would be deafness in one ear and tinnitus. On my life path, a personal setback with the loss of my career.

Q: If you could write a motto, what would it say?

A: One step at a time on the road to recovery. Expect to make a few stops along the way, but you will get there.

Q: If you had five pieces of advice to share?

A: The first is don't be tempted to rush for 'cures' as soon as you are diagnosed. The second: Don't try to 'quick fix' with surgery. The third: Realize there is a lot you can do to help yourself get over Meniere's. The fourth: Practice a modicum of patience. It can take some time to make a recovery and it doesn't happen overnight. But it does happen. The fifth: Don't give up hope.

Q: What advice can you give to conquer fear?

A: Fear comes from the unknown. Get the facts. Get answers to your questions. Voice your fears. Talk to people you trust. Getting emotional support from others can help dissipate fear.

Q: What is one personal attribute essential for recovery?

A: Determination to achieve the goal of recovery.

Q: What does health mean to you nowadays?

A: True success in life.

Q: How would you define good health?

A: Good health is not just about the lack of disease. Good health means complete physical, social and mental well-being.

Q: What is more important to you? Health or wealth?

A: At one stage in my life, I thought money was most important. I didn't pay that much attention to health. I left health to take care of itself. Having been through Meniere's, I'd say, health is the true wealth.

Q: What is your thought on conquering Meniere's?

A: Don't accept what you cannot control.

Q: What thing do you know about Meniere's for sure?

A: Prosper Meniere discovered it. Everything else is experiential.

Q: *What was the most serious illness you've had to face?*

A: *So far in my life, it has been Meniere's. If I ever find myself with another serious disease or illness, I will apply the same self-help and mindful recovery principles as I did for Meniere's disease. The four main aims are the same: to cope, to get healthier, to get better —to make a full recovery.*

Q: *How different now are you than before Meniere's?*

A: *I have more belief in the body's own ability to heal itself, with positive thinking and by doing as much for your health as you can. The power the mind plays in healing the body, never ceases to amaze me.*

Q: *What personal habits did you break?*

A: *The habit of multi-tasking to excess. I stopped stacking one activity on to another, all day, every day.*

Q: *Was Meniere's a traumatic event?*

A: *Yes it was a totally unexpected life-changing event.*

Q: *What character trait did Meniere's change?*

A: *I was a man of action. I did everything for myself and others and more. It was difficult to put myself first in the life equation, but I just had to adopt an attitude of self-preservation. I learned to say No without feeling guilty about* *that simple two letter word. NO!*

Q: *Was there ever a time when you thought you'd die?*

A: *No, never. Although there were days when I almost wished I could!*

Q: *What was the hardest era of your life?*

A: *My time negotiating the mountain of Meniere. I stumbled on all of its stones. It was an uphill battle and a test of personal endurance and strength at times.*

Q: *What do you think was a Meniere's epiphany?*

A: *Seeing the connection between triggers and attacks. Understanding that relationship was the turning point. I armed myself with personal facts to begin to counter the vertigo attacks.*

Q: *Before Meniere's was your glass half empty or half full?*

A: *It was half full, for sure.*

Q: *What was the most significant loss you had?*

A: *A feeling of confidence and 'joie de vivre'. The enjoyment of everything in life was difficult, because symptoms have a way of stealing happiness.*

Q: *Why do you think you had Meniere's?*

A: I think Meniere's showed up with work stress over a long period of time.

Q: Did you feel like you were merely existing or living?

A: Honestly when I had Meniere's, I felt a shadow of myself, just going through routines and trying to get through each day. It wasn't my choice. That was the hard part. For me, living a full life is about having freedom of choice. Meniere's is a dictator and a tough taskmaster. Meniere's takes your choice away. You can't live life without considering Meniere's. But once you take control back and start to manage your symptoms, Meniere's will stop managing you. That point marks the beginning of living your life again.

Q: How did you make peace with yourself?

A: Acceptance. This was key and very important. I stopped fighting Meniere's. I accepted I had the condition. The more I accepted the condition, the more I could do to help myself.

Q: How did Meniere's fuel impetus?

A: Meniere's was a cathartic experience. Overcoming a life hurdle of such magnitude, provided an opportunity to understand that many things in life are possible, no matter what people may say. Overcoming the impossible really is possible if you set your mind to it.

Q: What lessons did illness teach you?

A: Good old-fashioned moderation and discipline. Also to truly listen to my body and pay attention to intuition.

Q: If you were diagnosed over again what would you do?

A: I would start management on day one. I wouldn't waste a day. There is a lot you can do to help yourself. Focus on getting your body healthy. Make proactive lifestyle changes: exercise, diet, supplements, stress relief. Through every day, no matter what Meniere's throws at you, strive to keep a positive attitude.

Q: What did you manage to achieve with Meniere's?

A: I managed to understand my Meniere's, work out how to cope with symptoms and get better.

Q: What positives have resulted from your experience?

A: The virtual elimination of everything that appeared negative or harmful to me, both emotionally and physically.

Q: How do you comfort someone who is suffering?

A: Trust that your body will constantly work to get better until you are better, if you allow and enable your body to heal.

Q: How is life after Meniere's for you?

A: Life with Meniere's and life without Meniere's are poles apart. I was given a hopeless prognosis of an incurable disease for life, but it certainly wasn't the case. Once I recovered from Meniere's, I felt like I got my old life back again —and much more. I was a lot healthier. Now, I'm not only free of Meniere's, but I snowboard, ski, surf, hike and travel. I can work on my computer for hours. In short, I am back living a full and active life. If you saw me years ago, when Meniere's controlled every waking moment —I struggled to get out of bed.

Q: Do you have a 'Bucket List?'

A: Yes, for sure! Don't we all? Time stops for no one. No matter how much you make plans, you can never predict how life will go. Suffering from Meniere's took a chunk of time away from me. My calendar is full and I am not wasting a day of it.

REFERENCES

American Academy of Otolaryngology-Head and Neck Surgery's 1995
Guidelines for the Diagnosis and Evaluation of Therapy in Meniere's disease.
AAO- HNS: American Academy of Otolaryngology and Head and Neck Surgery; PTA: Pure Tone Audiometry; DHI: Dizziness Handicap Inventory

American Academy of Otolaryngology-Head and Neck Foundation, Inc.(1995). "Committee on Hearing and Equilibrium guidelines for the diagnosis and evaluation of therapy in Meniere's disease. " Otolaryngol Head Neck Surg 113(3): 181-185.

Anderson JP, Harris JP. Impact of Meniere's disease on quality of life. Otol Neurotol 22:888-894,2001

HAVIA M, Kentala E. Progression of symptoms of dizziness in Meniere's disease. Arch Otolaryngol Head Neck Surg 2004;130:431-5.

Honrubia V. Pathophysiology of Meniere's disease. Meniere's Disease (Ed. Harris JP) 231-260, 1999, Pub: Kugler (The Hague)

Huppert, D., et al. (2010). "Long-term course of Meniere's disease revisited." Acta Otolaryngol 130(6): 644-651.

MATEIJSEN DJ, Van Hengel PW, Van Huffelen WM, Wit HP, Albers FW. Pure-tone and speech audiometry in patients with Meniere's disease. Clin Otolaryngol 2001; 26: 379-87.

Santos, P. M., R. A. Hall, et al. (1993). "Diuretic and diet effect on Meniere's disease evaluated by the 1985

Committee on Hearing and Equilibrium guidelines." Otolaryngol Head Neck Surg 109(4): 680-9.

Savastino M, Marioni G, Aita M. Psychological characteristics of patients with Meniere's disease compared with patients with vertigo, tinnitus or hearing loss. ENT journal, 148-156, 2007

Savastano M, Maron MB, Mangialaio M, Longhi P, Rizzardo R. Illness behavior, personality traits, anxiety and depression in patients with Meniere's disease. J Otolaryngol 1996 Oct;25(5):329-333.

Sato G1, Sekine K, Matsuda K, Ueeda H, Horii A, Nishiike S, Kitahara T, Uno A, Imai T, Inohara H, Takeda N. Long-term prognosis of hearing loss in patients with unilateral Ménière's disease.Acta Otolaryngol. 2014 Jul 16:1-6. [Epub]

Soto-Varela A1, Huertas-Pardo B, Gayoso-Diz P, Santos-Perez S, Sanchez-Sellero I. Disability perception in Ménière's disease: when, how much and why? Eur Arch Otorhinolaryngol. 2015 May 1. [Epub]

Stahle J, Friberg U, Svedberg A. Long-term progression of Meniere's disease. Acta Otolaryngol (Stockh) 1991:Suppl 485:75-83

Jules Renard www.brainyquote.

Resource.nlm.gov

medicinenet.com/caffeine/article htm

Coping with chronic illness www.alpineguild.com

Hearing Loss - Merck Manuals Professional Edition.

Thirlwall, A. S. and S. Kundu (2006). "Diuretics for Meniere's disease or syndrome." Cochrane Database Syst Rev 3: CD003599.

"Ménière's Disease." The Alternate Advisor: The Complete Guide to Natural Therapies and Alternative Treatments. Edited by Robert. Richmond, VA: Time-Life Books, 1997

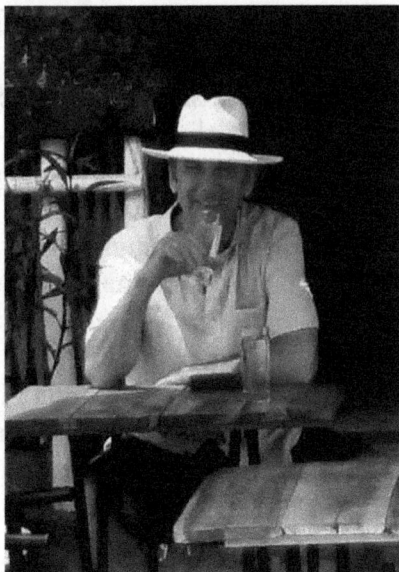

ABOUT MENIERE MAN

The Author is a writer, painter and designer. He is married to a Poet, and they have two adult children. He spends his time writing and painting. He loves the sea, nature, cooking, travel and the company of family, friends and his beloved dog Bella.

If you enjoyed this book and you think it may be helpful to others, please leave a review for this book.

MENIERE MAN BOOKS

MENIERE'S #1 BEST SELLER 3RD EDITION

MENIERE MAN
MAKE A FULL RECOVERY

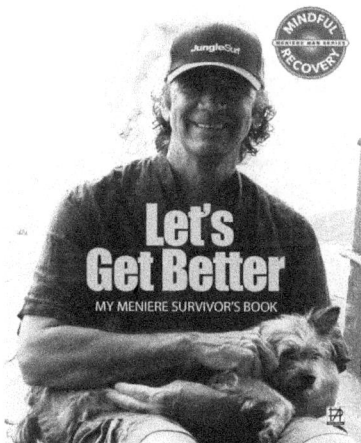

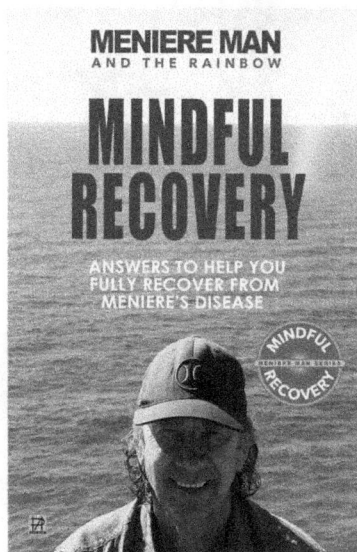

MINDFUL RECOVERY

Let's Get Better
MY MENIERE SURVIVOR'S BOOK

MENIERE MAN
AND THE RAINBOW

MINDFUL RECOVERY

ANSWERS TO HELP YOU
FULLY RECOVER FROM
MENIERE'S DISEASE

MINDFUL RECOVERY

MENIERE MAN
AND THE ASTRONAUT

THE
SELF-HELP
BOOK FOR
MENIERE'S
DISEASE

MINDFUL
RECOVERY

It's the only positive, yet real account
I've read, of what it's really like.
- L. Forrester.(UK)

MENIERE MAN
AND THE FILM DIRECTOR

THE
SELF-HELP
BOOK FOR
MENIERE'S
VERTIGO

MINDFUL
RECOVERY

"After I discovered how to manage
the Beginning, Middle and End stages
of acute vertigo, **I never suffered
another vertigo attack.**"
-Meniere Man

PAGE ADDIE PRESS
UNITED KINGDOM

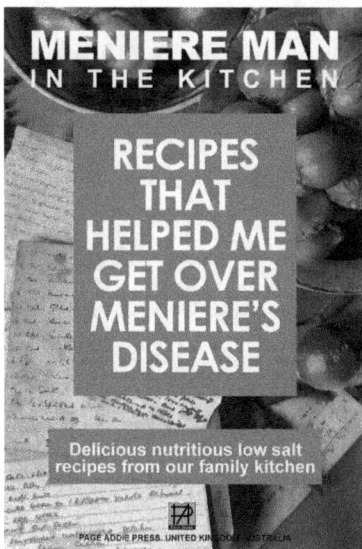

MENIERE MAN
IN THE KITCHEN

RECIPES
THAT
HELPED ME
GET OVER
MENIERE'S
DISEASE

Delicious nutritious low salt
recipes from our family kitchen

PAGE ADDIE PRESS, UNITED KINGDOM, AUSTRALIA

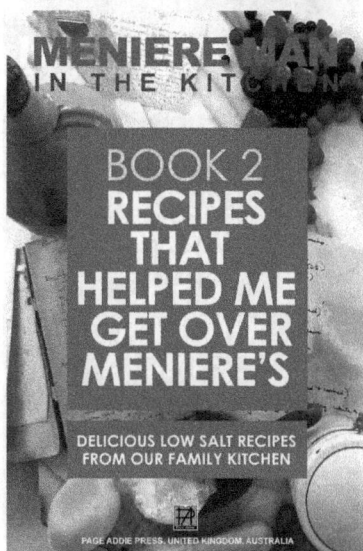

MENIERE MAN
IN THE KITCHEN

BOOK 2
RECIPES
THAT
HELPED ME
GET OVER
MENIERE'S

DELICIOUS LOW SALT RECIPES
FROM OUR FAMILY KITCHEN

PAGE ADDIE PRESS, UNITED KINGDOM, AUSTRALIA

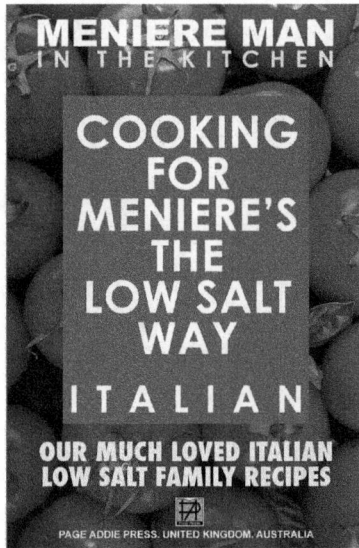

MENIERE MAN
IN THE KITCHEN

COOKING
FOR
MENIERE'S
THE
LOW SALT
WAY

ITALIAN

OUR MUCH LOVED ITALIAN
LOW SALT FAMILY RECIPES

PAGE ADDIE PRESS. UNITED KINGDOM. AUSTRALIA

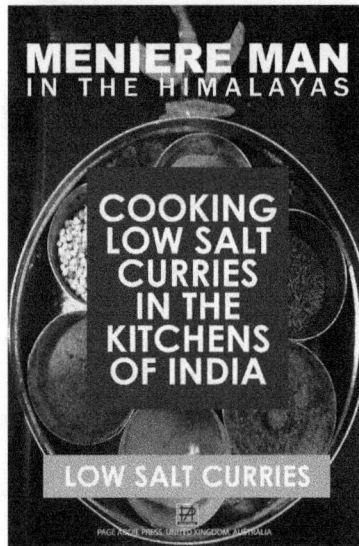

MENIERE MAN
IN THE HIMALAYAS

COOKING
LOW SALT
CURRIES
IN THE
KITCHENS
OF INDIA

LOW SALT CURRIES

PAGE ADDIE PRESS. UNITED KINGDOM. AUSTRALIA

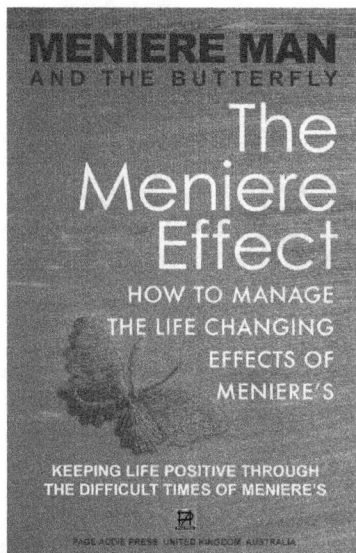

MENIERE MAN
AND THE BUTTERFLY

The
Meniere
Effect

HOW TO MANAGE
THE LIFE CHANGING
EFFECTS OF
MENIERE'S

KEEPING LIFE POSITIVE THROUGH
THE DIFFICULT TIMES OF MENIERE'S

PAGE ADDIE PRESS. UNITED KINGDOM. AUSTRALIA.

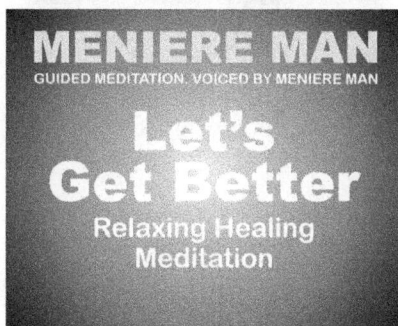

MENIERE MAN
GUIDED MEDITATION. VOICED BY MENIERE MAN

Let's
Get Better
Relaxing Healing
Meditation

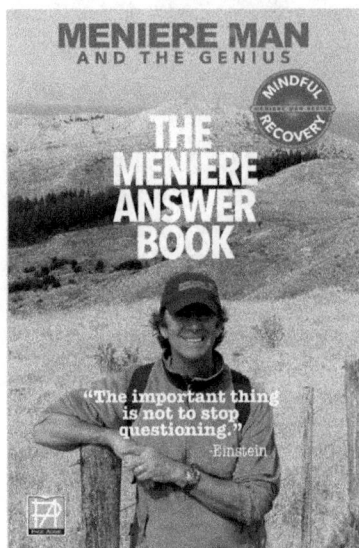

MENIERE MAN
AND THE GENIUS

MINDFUL
RECOVERY

THE
MENIERE
ANSWER
BOOK

"The important thing
is not to stop
questioning."
-Einstein

www.ingramcontent.com/pod-product-compliance
Lightning Source LLC
Chambersburg PA
CBHW060318030426
42336CB00011B/1100